WHAT'S UP WITH
MY HAIR?

WHAT'S UP WITH MY HAIR?

A practical guide to tackling the root cause of
alopecia areata & diffuse hair loss.

By Mary Corrigan

What's Up With My Hair?

Before embarking on either of the food plans you should consult your doctor to ensure that the menus and supplements are suitable for you, particularly if you are taking any medication or have any medical condition.

While the author has made every effort to ensure that the information given is as up to date and accurate as possible, it is based on her own experience and should be advisory only and not used as an alternative to specialist medical advice. The author and publisher cannot be held responsible for actions that may be taken by a reader as a result of reliance on the information contained in this book, which are taken entirely at the reader's own risk.

Copyright © Mary Corrigan 2010

First edition April 2011

Published by
What's Up With My Hair Publishing
52 Ashgrove Road, Bromley BR1 4JW

Mary Corrigan has asserted her moral right to be identified as the author of this work in accordance with the Copyright, Designs and Patents Act, 1998.

Cover design by Matt Gray

ISBN 978-0-9568262-0-6

Printed and bound by CPI Antony Rowe Limited, Chippenham

Acknowledgements

I would like to thank everyone who helped me through my hair loss days and who in turn, supported and encouraged me whilst writing this book.

Many thanks to Caroline, for tending my locks when my hair was at its worst and who also had a coffee ready whenever I was feeling down. Thanks also to Linda who was always at the end of the phone for many a reassuring chat.

I would like to thank my parents, brother and his family who were all unwavering in their support, even when I hit rock bottom, along with countless other family and friends.

To my daughters, Enya, Jessica and Caitlin, they will never know how uplifting their reassurances were when they would tell me it really didn't matter if I had hair or not, I was still their mummy.

Finally the biggest thanks must go to my ever tolerant husband Mark, who never once allowed my hair loss and the associated complications have any impact on our wonderful marriage.

Introduction

Over a period of two years I suffered the stress and turmoil of seeing my once fine head of hair, being reduced to virtual baldness. Each time I had a "grow back" period I was elated, when the shedding returned (each cycle producing ever larger patches) I was devastated. Dealing with the psychological aspect of hair loss became an uphill struggle as with every handful of hair shed, another aspect of my identity seemed to go with it. The person reflected in the mirror, was not the person I had known for 40 years!

The aim of this book is to try and help other women in potentially similar circumstances, eliminate months of worry and "not knowing". By following a step by step approach to your hair loss, perhaps we can help identify the cause or trigger of your Telogen Effluivium (excessive hair shedding) and/or Alopecia Areata (bald patches in varying sizes).

When I was not happy with the initial response from my doctor's surgery in diagnosing and treating my hair loss, I took it upon myself to try and work out what was going on inside my body. I am fortunate in that I have been able to invest many hours into researching the potential causes for my hair loss and then following the requisite treatment. I appreciate that many women in similar situations may not have the time and/or resources to do the same, which is why I want to share my findings. In addition I was able to use the Chef's skills and nutritional knowledge I acquired many years ago, whilst devising the food plans.

I have to stress at this point that I am not a medical practitioner and if anyone reading this book wants to follow suggestions made, they should check with their GP/Doctor first. Also, as the information provided is based on my own experience, there are aspects of Alopecia that I do not touch on such as how it affects men and children.

There are several good books available that can tell you all about the intricacies of the condition Alopecia. However, my aim is to provide practical advice such as knowing which blood tests to request from your GP/Doctor, which supplements to take to enhance hair growth and a diet plan to follow to either boost iron levels or kill off candida in the gut, as both conditions are known to cause hair loss.

A fountain of knowledge is useful, but you need to be focussing your energies on tackling the cause of your hair loss. I cannot guarantee that we will resolve your hair loss, but I can guarantee that you will feel a whole lot better both physically and mentally for trying!

Contents

CHAPTER 1

My Hair Loss Experience

When my dramatic hair loss began I was a 39 year old woman, married with three children and if you asked anyone over the period of my lifetime to describe me, I can guarantee the first thing they would mention is my hair. "Red", "thick", "curly", "long" were all words commonly associated with describing my crowning glory. On more than one occasion my hair has been described as my "defining feature". Not any more. For over a two year period my hair had been falling out.

It started with two small patches of alopecia, followed a few months later by a major bout of diffuse hair loss (Telogen Effluvium), followed once again by a much more severe attack of Alopecia Areata, resulting in ever increasing large, bald patches which eventually joined together leaving me practically bald.

At the time of starting this book, I was sitting at the computer predominantly bald, but for a few longer strands on the back of my head and a stubbly, patchy re-growth on the top. Four months later, I had established a really good coverage of thick strong hair. If you did not know me, you would assume I had a short hair style.

I have suffered alopecia areata twice before. When I was eighteen taking my A levels, I discovered a bald patch about the size of a 5p piece on the back of my head. My GP diagnosed it as being stress related. The second time was when I was twenty five and a couple of weeks before I got married. Again, stress was diagnosed as the cause. At the time these diagnoses seemed to make sense, however, I now have a different theory which I will go into later on.

Fast forward fourteen years to May 2006 and I discovered a familiar round patch on the back of my head. A few days later a second patch appeared and not long after a third. I went to my Doctor's surgery and was diagnosed with alopecia areata, once again, due to stress. My husband had been through a period of unemployment and although he was settled in a new job, the GP explained that it was a delayed reaction to the stressful time we had been through. He ordered a Full Blood Count blood test which came back normal, thus supporting this theory.

I decided this was an opportune time to make a concerted effort to get myself in better physical shape and started a period of strict but healthy eating, accompanied by a rigorous exercise routine. In October we went on a family holiday to Florida USA, during which I discovered a couple more small patches. I had my hair cut shorter as I though it would make it more manageable. However, by mid-November the hair loss had resumed, but instead of the classic small circular patches, it was coming out by the handful (otherwise known as diffuse hair loss). I mentioned it to my hairdresser who noticed a marked decline in the volume of my hair and she suggested I went back to my GP.

This time I saw a different Doctor. Once again I was asked about my home life and was told that the stress of every day life, raising three young children was taking its toll and I should try relaxing at a regular yoga class. I walked out of the surgery unconvinced. Three years earlier I had suffered a very difficult pregnancy, contracted an MRSA infection in the caesarean wound from my daughter's delivery, was subjected to verbal abuse by staff in the hospital and this was compounded by my husband being made redundant 2 weeks later! If this was not a stress inducing situation (that did not result in any hair loss) what was!!!

In addition to the hair loss I started suffering other symptoms. Extreme lethargy, weight gain, lowered body temperature, feeling cold and forgetfulness, to name but a few. My once thick hair which I used to struggle to tie up with a large elastic scrunchy, was reduced to a pathetic pony tail, barely the thickness of a pencil.

Researching my symptoms led me to suspect I was suffering from hypothyroidism (underactive thyroid gland). After a particularly upsetting hair washing session, my husband took control of the situation and took me up to the emergency surgery, armed with photographs showing my hair loss over the previous 6 months. We saw yet a different GP, but this time got a much more positive response. She was concerned about the marked hair loss and ordered a ream of blood tests including, Full Blood Count, Thyroid Function, Lupus and hormone levels to assess if I was starting an early menopause. I left this appointment feeling very positive however, a week later when all the test results were normal I felt utter despair when the now familiar "stress related" diagnosis was given. I was referred to a Homeopathic Doctor to see if this could help the condition in any way.

With hair still falling out by the handful I decided to take some positive action myself. Initially I decided the logical thing to research was "what makes healthy hair grow?" After a few hours on the internet, having ploughed through all the sites selling magical pills and potions, I compiled a list of vitamins, minerals and nutrients required for healthy hair. I informed my GP that this was the path I was taking and at this stage I was told that although my haemoglobin count was within the "normal" range, it was right at the bottom of it.

Over the next twelve weeks I religiously took iron, L-lysine, vitamins C, B6, B12, magnesium and zinc on a daily basis, ensuring they were spaced correctly throughout the day, before meals etc to ensure maximum impact. For the first few weeks the hair loss continued, but it then started to slow up and stop. After three months I discontinued taking the supplements in the belief that they had solved the problem. By my 40th birthday in March I felt up to facing a few close friends to celebrate. Although I had to have my hair cut short for the first time in 25 years, it looked good. The shedding had stopped, the patches, although shorter, had filled in and healthier hair was growing. I felt I had turned a corner and looked forward to putting the past twelve months behind me.

Then three months later (June 2007) I felt the dreaded patch on top of my head whilst washing my hair. A few days later another one started and I felt sick. I went back to my GP and she agreed to test my thyroid function again, but the result came back as "plum" normal. This meant I was right in the centre of the accepted range and therefore it was not possible to be suffering from hypothyroidism. My GP had this confirmed by an Endocrinologist. As the summer went on the hair loss got worse. Whereas before I was able to disguise large patches on the back of my head with longer layers of hair, this time I had no such luxury.

I hit the internet again and found research that backed up my theory of using the supplements and iron tablets. This time a particular piece of research I found, stated that women who used this supplement regime to get their hair back in shape, often found that within three months of stopping the regime, they started losing hair again. I was text book!

However, I also learned that it was my serum ferritin level that needed to be checked. Serum ferritin can show how low your body's iron stores are. It is a very important test to have when determining your iron levels as you can have low serum ferritin, but a normal haemoglobin level in your blood. This is because your body is depleting your iron stores for red blood cell production and the stores are not being topped up. Eventually there is no iron left to be drawn on and this is when you become anaemic. I thought this sounded logical, although I still suspected I was suffering from hypothyroidism as none of the other symptoms had gone away.

My GP was concerned that the hair loss had resumed and sent me for further blood tests in August, this time including serum ferritin. My regular tests came back as normal, but my serum ferritin level was nineteen, indicating very low iron stores. Some research states that if your levels are under 40, it is highly likely you may start losing hair. However, Philip Kingsley, a well known Trichologist, recently reported that levels need to be at a minimum of 80 nanograms of ferritin per millilitre (ng/ml) for hair follicles to function optimally. Any levels under 80ng/ml require medical intervention in the form of iron tablets, as it is unlikely you would be able to boost your iron stores significantly by diet alone. My GP set a target of 150, as the normal range goes up to 290.

We discussed which form of iron I should use. I opted for elemental iron over ferrous sulphate this time, as it is supposed to be absorbed into the body easier and is much gentler on the stomach. Unfortunately, it is not available on the NHS, so I had to purchase it privately. I also resumed taking the other vitamins and minerals which I had taken in the past.

Two months later when I returned to my GP for another test of my serum ferritin level, she was shocked to see how much hair I had lost. Hair growth on my body had also slowed up. This was apparent when I went for a six weekly leg wax appointment and my therapist commented on how little re-growth there had been. In addition my eyebrows were thinning. Whilst my serum ferritin level had increased to 37, I was still under the magical "40" and consequently, had lost so much hair by this stage, I was practically bald. She arranged an emergency consultation with a Dermatologist and the appointment came through four weeks later. By the time I attended the appointment, my hair had started its "grow back" phase again. I explained to the Dermatologist that I was now in a pattern of alopecia patches developing and re-growing, but each time I started a new pattern of hair loss, the patches were getting bigger and bigger until the current worst attack, where they all joined up together

The Dermatologist effectively confirmed what I had suspected at this stage. That low iron stores was the root of the problem. Particularly as the hair loss resumed three months after ceasing the iron and vitamin regime earlier in the year. She said that although I was building my iron stores throughout the month, a lot would be lost through the menstrual cycle. Indeed it was probable that this problem had been building over many years, before finally culminating last year.

After the birth of my first two daughters I was diagnosed as anaemic, due to haemorrhaging during delivery. With my first daughter I was offered a blood transfusion which I declined because the blood loss was not life threatening and I opted to rebuild my levels with iron tablets. After the second birth I was anaemic again, but on this occasion, as it was a milder form, was given a month's supply of iron tablets. Finally, my third daughter was delivered by caesarean section so I was not surprised to find out that once again, I was anaemic and sent home with more iron tablets.

What the Dermatologist pointed out, was the fact that I did not have follow up blood tests to ensure that my iron levels had been re-established to a desirable level.

I was advised to continue taking iron tablets on a daily basis and that I would have to have my serum ferritin levels checked every three months, to ensure I was maintaining a reasonable level of iron. She said it was highly likely that this will be the case until I have gone through the menopause and my periods have ceased. (Although, I was told that medical intervention can be made to lower the level of menstrual loss, if necessary).

I left the appointment with mixed emotions. On the one hand I felt a huge relief with my hair loss being attributed to low iron levels and it was easily treatable. On the other hand I was annoyed that my family and I had to suffer the stress and emotional turmoil of the past eighteen months, when a simple blood test could have provided a potential diagnosis at the beginning. I appreciate that not all cases of alopecia areata will be caused by low iron stores. But for many women suffering the indignity of hair loss, they too could have their anguish diminished by a simple blood test, at least giving them an avenue of treatment to try.

Throughout this whole process, even with a diagnosis from the Dermatologist, no-one has offered advice on how to bolster my iron stores through dietary means. I have conducted extensive research to find out how to eat an effective, iron rich diet. I say effective, because there are many factors that will affect the uptake of iron by the body. I eventually devised an Iron Rich Booster Plan in an attempt to bolster my iron intake as much as possible (See Chapter 7).

It was only later that I was to realise that although low iron levels can be responsible for diffuse hair loss, research does not appear to support it being a factor in Alopecia Areata. However, once again I resumed the iron, vitamin & supplement regime. By Christmas I would not go out in public without a hat, but at least my whole head was covered in approximately two centimetres of hair.

Then on New Year's Day 2008 my husband noticed a small patch on the top of my head. Once again, that familiar feeling of nausea and dread rose up within me. Was I ever going to be shot of this debilitating condition?

I returned to the GP and asked for another serum ferritin blood test. I was shocked at the result. The level was 38. So I had gone up by 1ng since October! Something was not right. I asked my GP if she could start a new line of investigation. Why was I not absorbing iron? Although I was assured that this was not necessary, as I had been tested for this previously, I was not convinced. The only option available was to consider going on the pill to reduce my menstrual flow. Again, I was not keen as I did not get on with the pill years ago and did not want to put more drugs into my body, until I knew what was going on.

Although I was upset by the set back, it did confirm the niggling doubt at the back of my mind, that the alopecia was a symptom of another unidentified problem. I recalled the previous occasions when I experienced alopecia and tried to establish some form of link.

The only thing I could come up with was on both previous occasions, I had been given high doses of antibiotics in the run up to the hair loss.

I recalled that during my mid-twenties I contracted a serious viral infection and was hospitalised for a week, on an isolation ward, being pumped intravenously with antibiotics. A few months later I was diagnosed with Myalgic Encephalomyelitis (ME) more recently known as Chronic Fatigue Syndrome. At the time, in desperation, I saw an Applied Kinesiologist. Although sceptical about the way in which these practitioners operate, I was diagnosed in the first session as suffering from Candida of the small intestine and leaky gut. The Practitioner said my immune system had been compromised, due to the high volume of antibiotics destroying the "good" bacteria in my gut. This in turn allowed the candida to grow and spread, with the side effects presenting as extreme lethargy, aching and swollen joints, food intolerances, unexplained weight gain, to name but a few symptoms. However, I completely recovered within six weeks after following a strict diet to "kill" the candida. In addition I took supplements to replace the vitamins and minerals I had been diagnosed as being deficient in and finally a good probiotic, acidophilus, to replace the "good" bacteria in my gut.

I decided that it would be worth my while to seek the opinion of an Applied Kinesiologist, in relation to my hair loss.

During the consultation, the practitioner did identify that my iron levels were lower than usual, but did not consider this to be the current cause of my hair loss. He said it was likely that my body was having difficulty absorbing iron, because iron is absorbed in the small intestine and he identified that my small intestine was overrun with candida, hence making the absorption of all nutrients difficult. He also diagnosed a leaky gut. This is where the valve from the small intestine does not close properly and therefore allows waste products to "back up" into the small intestine. Most importantly he advised me that this condition can result in hair loss. As the gut had been taken over with the candida, despite following a healthy diet, very little nutrition was being absorbed. Consequently the hair loss commenced as the hair is one of the first places the body can deprive of nutrition, without having a major detrimental effect on the overall functioning of the body.

In February 2008 I started an "Anti Candida" food plan. At this stage patches of hair were approximately two inches long. But new bald patches were developing all the time. Once again I was caught in a hair loss cycle and if the previous event was anything to go by, my body would not stop until I was bald again!

I found the diet difficult to begin with as I had been given the guidelines, but had to devise a whole new diet for myself.

An Anti-Candida diet entails eliminating ALL forms of sugar. Apart from the obvious sources, you have to read labels very carefully as sugars can be disguised in many forms, primarily to act as a flavour enhancer. Anything ending in "ose", ie: sucrose, lactose is sugar. This also included fruit (with the exception of apples) and high sugar vegetables such as carrots. In addition I had to eliminate any food types that have been fermented such as vinegar and yeast products, as well as avoid fungal based vegetables – potatoes and mushrooms and avoid any foods with moulds, such as blue veined cheeses. I also had to be aware that nuts, if not fresh, can have minute formations of mould on them. Finally I had to give up alcohol, as this converts to sugar.

The reason for the severity of the food plan is to starve the candida of its life source. In addition to the food exclusions, I drank a herbal tincture called Bittersweet to aid the elimination of the candida and I also took the hair promoting supplements again.

During the six weeks that I followed the diet religiously, I also researched Candida. There are different schools of thought as to how long you should follow an Anti-Candida diet. Many suggest a minimum of three months. However, I believe that this relates to your own personal symptoms as Candida can present itself in many different forms, as I discovered in the past when I was diagnosed with ME. Also, every person is different and may take longer or shorter periods of time to not only eliminate the Candida from their body, but they may then be more susceptible to re-current attacks. I can only speak from my own experience and how it related to my hair loss.

I also discovered that low iron levels can stimulate the environment which Candida thrives on. As a fungus Candida will reproduce quicker when there is a lack of oxygen. Iron is responsible for enabling the red blood cells to carry oxygen around the body. If iron levels are low, then the cells of the body will not be receiving optimum oxygen levels. To increase the oxygen levels the body needs to absorb more iron and to achieve this, the Candida needs to be eliminated from the gut, to enable maximum absorption of iron, as well as all other nutrients.

I now know that my body cannot tolerate large doses of antibiotics, without side effects. It seems to take several months, even years for the candida to dominate my small intestine. However, it would appear to have the ability to wreak havoc with my health. On both occasions of receiving high dose intravenous antibiotics, I have suffered from firstly the debilitating condition, ME and secondly, the equally psychologically debilitating conditions of both diffuse hair loss and chronic alopecia areata.

As I said earlier, it took a lot of will power to stick to the diet. I had to keep remembering that the smallest amount of sugar within the given period could be enough to feed the candida and re-establish its growth.

During the six weeks I continued to lose hair and a couple of new patches developed. When the Practitioner re-tested me at this time, he said that the candida had gone, so I could start introducing the excluded foods into my diet again. I also started taking a good quality probiotic to re-establish good bacteria in my gut. This helps to reduce the chances of the candida taking a hold again, should it be re-introduced.

Once again, I felt that this line of investigation had failed, as I was still suffering hair loss. However, I was thrilled that the side effect of following the diet meant that I had lost a stone in weight. Because of the weight loss, I continued to follow the principles of the Anti-Candida diet, albeit in a more relaxed way. Then, two weeks later, I noticed that one of the longer standing bald patches (two months or more) had some hair growth in it. I started feeling around my head and was excited that I was feeling velvety hair growth in all of the patches, even the ones that were only a couple of weeks old!

This was the turning point for my battle with alopecia areata. For the first time in two years I felt I had actually conquered the condition that had plagued my life for so long.

Over the next few months my hair continued to grow and this time the hair growing back was in fabulous condition. It is soft and curly in fact it is back to the way it was before I had children. Over the past few years I had got used to the fact that it had lost its curl and was much coarser in texture. I had put these changes down to the aging process!

I am still very conscious of my hair and from time to time will run my fingers over my scalp, still not quite believing that those smooth little patches have not reappeared.

I also know that I have to be more proactive in managing my health to prevent a similar occurrence again. Although I do need to lose some more weight, it is still in the back of my mind what happened in the run up to our trip to Florida. Namely, following an intensive diet and exercise regime which in retrospect, appears to have been the trigger for the initial diffuse hair loss. However, thanks to Joanna Hall and her Walk Active Club, I have learned that I can exercise effectively and not suffer hair loss as a consequence. Despite Joanna's assurances, I was very nervous that the walking would cause my iron levels to fall and trigger hair loss. I needn't have worried! Using her unique walking technique, I have toned up, lost weight, am much fitter and have found my confidence returning. In May 2010 I took part in the London Moon Walk, a 26 mile walk around central London throughout the night, to raise money for Breast Cancer Awareness. I would not have achieved this without the support of Joanna's Walk Active Club so I can highly recommend it. Even if you are suffering from hair loss, you can pop on a hat or scarf and go out walking anytime.

When I recall my two earlier brushes with alopecia areata, namely when I was taking my A levels at the age of eighteen years and seven years later when I was getting married, stress was diagnosed as the cause. Although I will concede that stress was also likely to be a contributory factor, it was not the only one. I now believe the hair loss was more likely to be linked to the intensive dieting and exercise programmes I was also following at the time. I had a tendency to follow strict vegetarian regimes whilst dieting, yet cutting out animal proteins proved to be very detrimental. After all, hair is made of keratin which is predominantly protein!

Going forward, a more gentle approach to health must be taken. No more fad diets and a less aggressive form of exercise, such as the walking. Also, I have learned that if too much sugar is re-introduced into the diet, it is possible for candida to take a hold again. Although it is unlikely to develop to the same extent, particularly without the contributory factors of high doses of antibiotics, as a preventative course of action, I intend to follow the Anti-Candida Plan once a year.

CHAPTER 2

Hair Loss Check List

Do any of the following apply to you?

Have you received antibiotic treatment, regardless of ailment?

Do you suffer from anaemia or have done in the past?

Do you suffer from thrush?

Have you self medicated for thrush with over the counter preparations?

Are you on the Pill, have a contraceptive implant, or have in the past?

Have you given birth in the past couple of years?

Have you experienced a change in your menstrual cycle?

Have you been on a really strict diet and / or exercise regime in the past few months?

Have you experienced a severe emotional shock / trauma in the past few months?

Do you suffer from asthma, hayfever, eczema or any other allergies?

Do you have ridged or pitted nails?

Do you experience scalp pain?

If you have said 'yes' to one or more on the above list, then you need to start eliminating possible causes for your hair loss. The above list could include possible triggers, but are not necessarily the cause, therefore look at the following list and see if you suffer from any of the following:
(it may be useful to highlight any symptoms that are applicable to you)

Fatigue	Depression	Sensitivity to cold	Weight gain
Forgetfulness	Dry skin	Dry hair	Constipation
Muscle cramps	Increased menstrual flow	Change in hair texture	Elevated cholesterol
Poor concentration	Recurrent infections	Muscle ache	Joint pain
Enlarged tongue	Thinning eyebrows	Thinning eyelashes	Slow pulse
Low blood pressure	Low body temperature (below 98.6c)	Muscle cramps	Heartburn

Dark circles under the eyes

Tongue symptoms including a line down the centre, teeth marks, yellowy coating and / or swelling

Once again, symptoms on the second list do not necessarily lead to the cause of your hair loss, but it can assist your GP in making an initial diagnosis. For example: several of the symptoms could indicate hypothyroidism (underactive thyroid), where hair loss is a common side effect. Whereas other symptoms are more likely to indicate anaemia or low iron stores such as dark circles under the eyes being a possible indicator in women. Ironically, low iron stores can mimic the symptoms of hypothyroidism, as can the overgrowth of candida in the gut.

CHAPTER 3

Doctors' Appointment

Once you have identified your symptoms, book an appointment with your Doctor to discuss your hair loss. It is quite likely that you will be told that your hair loss is probably the result of some form of stress in your life and this is possible. However, what you need to do is eliminate other possible causes, so please have a look at Chapter 14 first to see if you are taking any of the medications mentioned which may account for your hair loss.

When you go to the appointment, take with you a list of your symptoms and request the following blood tests to try and ascertain the possible cause of your hair loss.

1) Thyroid Activity (to assess the possibility of particularly Hypothyroidism but Hyperthyroidism can also cause hair loss)
2) Hormone Levels (to assess the possibility of Menopause)
3) Lupus (hair loss is a common symptom whilst Lupus is in an active phase)
4) Anaemia (low iron levels can cause hair loss)
5) Serum Ferritin Level (should ideally be above 80ng/ml)
   As a matter of course your GP may well want to check your vitamin B6/B12 levels, as well as other minerals.

Other diseases that can cause hair loss that your Doctor may discuss with you include Ringworm (fungal infection), Diabetes, Anorexia and Bulimia.

Check with your Doctor that you can take the following supplements to help support the healthy growth of hair: L-lysine, magnesium, zinc, selenium, vitamins B6 & B12, vitamin C.

If your GP agrees, then read the section on how to get the optimum benefit from your supplements.

If it transpires you are suffering from any of the first three ailments, your GP will be able to guide you through the required treatment and hopefully the re-growth of your hair will follow in due course. If you are still losing hair a few months after treatment commences, check with your GP if it is safe for you to try the Anti-Candida Plan, without it being detrimental to any medical treatment you are receiving.

If it transpires your hair loss is possibly related to low iron levels, your GP will prescribe you with a course of iron tablets. In this case, please read the section on iron deficiency as I have included tips on how to best absorb iron and have also included some iron rich recipes. Your GP should also investigate the cause of your low iron levels as there are numerous other ailments to the ones already mentioned which can result in the loss of blood from the body. These can include internal bleeding from gastritis and ulcers, inflammatory bowel disease, parasitic infections and haemorrhoids.

On commencing treatment with iron tablets you should book an appointment for three months time to request a further Serum Ferritin blood test, to ensure that your levels are increasing to an acceptable level. If after three months your levels are still low and you are struggling to raise them, please look at the Candida section and consider doing the Anti Candida Plan. It is possible that you have a Candida infection of the gut which is hindering the absorption of iron, vitamins and minerals required for healthy hair.

Finally, should all your test results come back normal, you can always request a referral to a Dermatologist. My referral came eighteen months after the initial diagnosis and I now believe it should have happened a lot earlier. My GP also referred me to a Homeopathic Doctor. I found this very interesting as a holistic approach to treating the symptoms, but ultimately homeopathy did not halt my hair loss.

Regardless of the next step your GP decides to take, still go to the Candida section of this book. It is quite possible that you are not absorbing sufficient nutrients to maintain healthy hair because of a Candida infection of the gut. If so, this is probably the easiest condition to treat, it just requires will-power to stick to the Anti-Candida Plan and hopefully, like me, you will see positive results.

CHAPTER 4

Supplements To Support Healthy Hair Growth & How To Include Them In Your Daily Diet

When I finally accepted that I had a problem with excessive hair shedding and alopecia areata, coupled with little advice on how to tackle this, my first thoughts were to look at what was required to establish healthy growth of hair.

Protein

This is essential in the diet as hair is predominantly made of keratin which is a form of protein. When we regularly do not eat sufficient quantities of protein to maintain the body's requirements, it is likely that the body, in an attempt to conserve protein for essential functions, will put hair follicles into resting phase prematurely, which will ultimately result in excessive shedding a few weeks later. So if you follow a strict diet for a few weeks you may not experience the side effects of it until AFTER you have come off it.

I do not recommend supplementing protein in any form other than a healthy diet. Have a look at the recipes in the Iron Boost Plan and Anti-Candida Plan to see examples of protein rich recipes.

Water

Sufficient intake of water will help to keep hair hydrated, supple and contribute towards keeping it silky and shiny. In fact water accounts for up to 25% of the weight of a strand of hair, so ensure you are drinking 1½ - 2 litres a day. If you are not used to consuming this volume of water, the easiest way to introduce it is to have a small glass every hour. Until your body gets used to the extra intake of water, you may initially be going to the loo more often, but this will settle down after a few days.

L-Lysine

This is an essential amino acid which plays a key part in the growth of hair. It is also often found to be in very low quantities in people suffering from low ferritin levels. Interestingly when a significant proportion of women on high iron and vitamin C intake failed to achieve the required ferritin levels, once L-Lysine supplements were added to the diet, most women went on to achieve their target ferritin levels and their hair volume subsequently increased. However, once the L-Lysine supplement was removed from the diet, hair shedding resumed several months later.

500mg L-Lysine Supplement – take twice a day, one in the morning with breakfast and one in the evening with dinner.

Vitamin C

This is responsible for the formation and maintenance of healthy collagen. Collagen is one of the proteins which constitutes to the make up of hair.

Vitamin C also helps with the absorption of iron in the diet. For this reason, if you are suffering from low iron levels, I would recommend a Vitamin C supplement.

100mg Vitamin C supplement – take three times a day, one with each meal.

Magnesium-B (manufactured by Wassen)

I have identified this particular supplement as it contains Magnesium, B complex vitamins, Folic Acid and Biotin. All are required for healthy hair growth and are provided in one tablet. This brand is readily available at chemists, pharmacies and health food stores.

Take one tablet per day.

Zinc & Selenium

These are both minerals that promote the healthy growth of hair. However too much of either mineral will cause hair loss. I did take a zinc supplement for a while (15mg per day), but I am going to suggest that you decide with your doctor whether or not you wish to add these supplements to the others suggested.

Aloe Vera Juice

Aloe Vera juice is very soothing and healing on the gut which is one of the reasons I recommend it.

Please be sure that you purchase it in its purest form (please see stockists list for suppliers) as it is now available with many different things added to it, such as sugar. I do not believe that the extra expense incurred for the added extras is necessary, particularly as you need to avoid sugar if you are following the Anti-Candida Plan.

Spirulina

I started taking Spirulina this year primarily to ensure that I am achieving a good daily intake of iron. Spirulina is an algae which is not only a very good source of iron, but also many of the daily vitamins, minerals and amino acids required for optimum health. I am currently using Hawaiian Spirulina (see suppliers list) as it is grown without herbicides or pesticides in Hawaii. It is also dried in a unique way to help preserve the nutritional values of the algae.

Spirulina is available in both tablet and powder form. I opted for powder, as I

14

did not want to take any more tablets. One teaspoon dissolved in orange juice gives you 6mg of iron. I take this once a day, although you can take it up to three times a day. This would be good to help boost your iron levels initially, however do remember that you should be trying to achieve a reasonable iron intake by following a balanced diet.

Take the Spirulina with orange juice as this provides the Vitamin C to help the absorption of the iron. Also, as with all other iron rich foods, ideally do not drink tea or coffee for an hour both before and after consumption, to ensure maximum absorption.

If you want to take Spirulina whilst following the Anti-Candida Plan, mix it with apple juice instead of orange juice to ensure you are not consuming the sugar found in oranges.

I followed the regime for three months and during that time, my hair grew back. However, after stopping the supplements, I resumed hair loss again within three months. Therefore, this indicated to me that the supplements were sufficient for my hair to grow, but without them I was not absorbing sufficient nutrition from my diet to maintain healthy hair. Hence my further studying the areas of low iron levels and Candidiasis influencing the body's ability to sustain hair.

Unless your Doctor has identified another probable cause, I suspect that your hair loss is most likely to be linked to either low iron stores and/or Candidiasis. Whilst you are attending to either or both of these conditions, your body is going to require some help in re-establishing optimum hair growth as quickly as possible. Please do not expect miracles. It will take a minimum of three months for you to reap the benefits of taking the supplements. Also, do not drop them as soon as you achieve re-growth.

If you have suffered from low serum ferritin levels, do not stop supplementation until you are near the 80ng/ml level. This may take six months or more.

If you suspect Candidiasis as the cause, continue with the supplements until you are confident that healthy hair re-growth has been established. Again, I would suggest three to six months.

Make a diary note of when you stop taking the supplements. If after three months your hair loss resumes, this would indicate that either your serum ferritin levels have dropped too low, or Candidiasis is re-established in the gut and you are not achieving sufficient absorption of nutrients.

CHAPTER 5

Preparations before commencing the Iron Rich Booster Plan and/or Anti Candida Plan

Before you embark on either of the plans I would suggest that firstly you read through the plan thoroughly and gain an understanding of how it may impact on your life. Perhaps you will require more preparation time in the kitchen, or maybe you will be using utensils and/or ingredients that you have not used before.

Please find listed below kitchen utensils that will be really handy to have available. If for example you do not possess a food processor and are cautious about buying one, perhaps you have a hand blender. This may take a little extra work, but I generally find it makes a good substitute. Alternatively, maybe you could borrow one from a family member, friend or neighbour.

Heavy based frying pan
Food processor &/or hand blender
Chopping board
Sharp knife
Wooden spoons
Plastic storage containers with lids for keeping ingredients in the fridge

Consider the timing of when you are going to start the plan. Try to avoid a hectic week so that you have the time to make any necessary adjustments to the way you shop, cook etcetera.

You may decide to ease your way into your selected plan over the period of a few days, to enable you to start breaking down any eating habits that will need to be adjusted.

For example: Start cutting back on your sugar intake and/or alcohol consumption if you are going to be following the Anti-Candida Plan.

Cooking With Oil.
You will probably note in the recipes that I use a variety of different oils and there is a reason for this. Contrary to long term health beliefs that oil is bad for you, using good oils in the correct proportions will give you optimum health benefits. These are the oils that I use and why I use them.

1. Linseed Oil – should only be used cold as heat will destroy the beneficial properties of the oil. Therefore it should be used in salad dressings and by adding 1 tablespoon to smoothie style drinks. Linseed oil is rich in Omega 3 so is excellent if you are watching your blood pressure and cholesterol levels. It also benefits the growth of hair and nails as well as numerous other benefits. For further information go to www.highbarnoils.co.uk.

2. Cold Pressed Rapeseed Oil – This oil can be heated and in fact, has a higher smoke point at 220 Centigrade than most other conventional cooking oils. It is also delicate in flavour so makes a great base for salad dressings. The main health benefits are the balance of the Omegas 3, 6 & 9 and that it contains half the saturated fat of olive oil.

3. Coconut Oil – comes in tubs and is solid when cold, but do not be put off by this. Coconut oil is a great anti-fungal and anti-bacterial so is ideal for use on the Anti-Candida Plan. It is also soothing on the gut, helps to balance cholesterol levels and increases immunity. It contains vitamins E & K as well as minerals including iron. In fact coconut oil has so many health benefits there are too many to mention here. Suffice it to say, being the cheapest of the oils mentioned so far, it may prove to be the best value for money. You can substitute any cooking oils on the plans with coconut oil although I would not suggest using it in salad dressings. It is also worth noting that this oil does not taint the food with a taste of coconut!

4. Olive Oil – I tend to use olive oil in the recipes that traditionally use it. There is a wide variety of qualities and flavours when it comes to olive oil. Extra virgin olive oil is purer and tends to have a stronger flavour. This is more expensive and not so good to cook with as regular olive oil, although it does make a good salad dressing. Olive oil has been proven as effective in reducing the build up of cholesterol and is also cited with inhibiting the growth of some cancers. It can also help to control blood sugar levels, which is of particular importance to people suffering from diabetes.

Look at the ingredients.
You may be introducing new food items that you have not eaten or prepared before. Please do not be put off by some of the recipes. When I first looked at some of my now favourite dishes such as fennel and cannellini beans or the use of puy lentils, I turned my nose up.

I strongly urge you to try everything at least once, then if you really do not like the dish, substitute it with an alternative. On the Iron Rich Plan look for an alternative with comparable iron levels as the one you wish to substitute out. Alternatively, you could boost your iron levels with an iron rich snack from the list provided.

On the Anti-Candida Plan, this serves to be more of a guide to ensure that you achieve a reasonably healthy pattern of eating, whilst excluding certain foods. Therefore, if you do not like a particular recipe substitute whatever you like, as long as you do not use any of the food types on the exclusion list.

Do not lose sight of why you are partaking of the eating plans. The fact that I may re-grow my hair whilst I was on the Anti-Candida Plan was what kept me going at my weakest points.

REMEMBER 1 teaspoon of sugar is enough to undo two - four weeks of work on the Anti-Candida Plan!

CHAPTER 6

Low iron levels and its influence on hair loss

Before commencing with this section, I feel it is important to make you aware that there is a disease caused by excessive iron in the blood. I want to make you aware of this condition, in case you are commencing this section without having had a full blood count or test of the level of your serum ferritin stores.

Haemochromatosis

This condition is caused by excessive iron levels in the body. Haemochromatosis can be a dangerous disease if undiagnosed as it affects the organs and can ultimately lead to organ failure. Haemochromatosis can be hereditary and can also be caused by the body destroying large numbers of abnormal blood cells and releasing their iron.

Haemochromatosis predominantly affects white populations at a rate of one in every 300 to 400 people, compared to black populations at half this rate. Men are more likely to suffer from it than women and it is especially prevalent in the Irish / Celtic populations.

In recent months there has been an advertisement on television for follow on milk for toddlers. It states that to take in the recommended 6mg of iron per day for a child of this age, they would have to drink twenty litres of cow's milk! Fortunately the follow on milk is fortified with iron and therefore a much more manageable quantity of 2 cups is required per day to fulfil the requirements. Unfortunately, as adults the majority of us are unaware of the importance of sufficient iron in our diet to maintain optimum health. Approximately 26% of the Western world (www.Florahealth.com) suffers from some form of iron deficiency and it can be responsible for many ailments. This is particularly pertinent to women as a certain amount of iron is lost per month through menstruation.

If you have suffered heavy shedding of hair, otherwise known as diffuse hair loss (Telogen effluvium), this could be due to having low iron levels in the body.

Iron is required for numerous functions within the body. It is necessary to make haemoglobin, the substance that carries oxygen through your blood to all of the cells in your body. If you do not have enough iron, then you may not produce sufficient haemoglobin, which in turn will mean that your red blood cells will not carry sufficient oxygen. This can sometimes be referred to as "tired blood" and if you have tired blood, you will have a tired body.

Iron is also needed for the brain. Neurotransmitters, the neurochemicals that carry the messages between nerves, require a sufficient level of iron to function properly. Low iron levels may well result in a tired mind (brain fog) as well as a tired body. Low iron levels will also impact on a healthy immune system and make you more susceptible to illness

Symptoms of low iron levels can include tiredness/fatigue, inflammation of the mouth and/or tongue, slow mental reactions, pale skin, ridged/pitted nails, lower body temperature, depression, rapid heartbeat, loss of libido and brittle hair, to name but a few!

Research has shown that a large proportion of women suffering from hair loss, also have low ferritin levels. This can be for a variety of reasons including the following:

Internal bleeding – blood loss due to bleeding from gastritis, ulcers, inflammatory bowel disease, parasitic infections and haemorrhoids.

Menstruation in women – iron is lost in the monthly period, particularly if the periods are heavy and last longer than four to five days.

Intensive or excessive exercise – particularly applies to long distance runners who are also prone to being low in calcium.

Diet – a high percentage of the population do not achieve the daily recommended level of iron in their diet. This is partly due to an increase in the use of processed foods, a reduction in the intake of red meat (particularly in the diet conscious who may consider it to be unhealthy) and a reduction in the consumption of leafy greens and legumes in the diet.

Negation of the consumption of iron – this means that the absorption of ingested iron can be radically reduced due to the consumption of iron absorption inhibitors at the same meal. For example: the tannins in tea or coffee will reduce the amount of iron you will absorb from your fortified breakfast cereal. Therefore tea and coffee should not be consumed for ideally 60 minutes before or after this meal. However, Vitamin C is widely known to maximise the absorption of iron and therefore, a glass of orange juice with your breakfast cereal is ideal.

The Environment - we are currently living in an environment where we are consuming more and more pre-prepared and processed foods. Therefore we are not always achieving our optimum nutritional requirements. I am sure we all have days when we do not achieve the Government recommendation of "five a day". This is not a problem if it occurs once in a while, but if this lifestyle is sustained over a long period of time, the effect of deficiencies can start to present themselves in numerous ways.

In addition a lot of food is now mass produced using intensive farming methods.

In his book "We Want Real Food", Graham Harvey details how the use of fertilisers, pesticides, hybrid seeds and over-farmed land have resulted in a depletion of essential minerals and nutrients in food. Essentially the nutrients that sustain healthy hair including iron, copper and zinc have been seriously affected. For example: Harvey talks about a comparative study of *The Composition of Foods (1991)* and a document published by the Medical Research Council in 1940. This study was undertaken by David Thomas, a geologist who also trained as a nutritionist. He discovered an alarming drop in the nutritional value of British fruit and vegetables during this time. He surmised that to gain the same amount of copper in a tomato from 1940, you would have to consume ten tomatoes in 1991!

Iron content alone had dropped by 46% in carrots, 45% in potatoes and as an average across all vegetables, an overall decrease of 27%.

Just as alarmingly in a range of ten popular cuts of meat, the iron levels had fallen by 54% and the copper content by 24%. I am assuming that this is due to the nutritional values in the animal feed having also decreased over the years.

These facts surely go some way towards explaining why, even if we are following a reasonable diet, so many people are now suffering from low levels of iron in their body. This makes it all the more important for us to consume the best food available to us within the confines of financial and time restrictions.

How do I find out if I have low Iron levels?

If you identify with the symptoms mentioned earlier, then you should ask your doctor for blood tests to see if you suffer from anaemia and most importantly, a test of your **Serum Ferritin Level** to identify if you have low iron stores.

The range for an acceptable Serum Ferritin is wide, but what you need to know is a level **below 40 nanograms of ferritin per millilitre (ng/ml)** is likely to cause hair loss and any level below 80ng/ml possibly requires treatment with iron tablets.

If your blood tests show that you require iron tablets then you should ensure that you are prescribed **ferrous sulphate** over ferric iron, as the body absorbs it easier. Another alternative to ferrous sulphate, which can have unpleasant side effects such as constipation, is **elemental iron**. This is much gentler on the stomach, but harder to acquire. I ordered mine from a recommended reputable company on the internet (please see suppliers list).

Please note: **Taking iron supplements that have not been prescribed by your GP can be extremely dangerous, as too much iron in the body can be harmful and cause irreversible damage. There are also other health conditions that can be adversely affected by iron tablets; so once again, your GP is the best person to advise you. DO NOT TAKE IT UPON YOURSELF TO SELF PRESCRIBE IRON TABLETS WITHOUT MEDICAL ADVICE.**

CHAPTER 7

Iron Rich Booster Plan

If you are prescribed iron supplements, then it is important that your iron levels are retested after a given period of time, usually three months, to ensure that you are absorbing it and have reached a desirable level. It is possible that three months will not be long enough, as it can take a while to rebuild iron stores within the body, so you may need to be retested after a further three months to ensure that your iron levels are increasing. However, it is possible to boost the process by eating an iron rich diet and learning how to best combine your foods to ensure maximum absorption of iron into the body.

Iron in your diet

This is not as straight forward as I initially thought it would be. I am of an age where I can remember watching cartoons of Popeye eating cans of spinach, full of iron, to support his bulging muscles. I was surprised to see that compared to other sources of iron rich foods spinach came low on the list. In addition, it is an iron absorption inhibitor which can *prevent* iron being absorbed.

Iron Absorption Inhibitors V Iron Absorption Enhancers

When I first learned about this subject area I threw my hands up in despair. All I wanted to do was boost my iron levels, yet it was proving to be so complicated!

For this reason, I have laid out my findings in a way which will hopefully enable you to get the optimum benefit from the iron rich foods you will consume.

Later I will provide an example of a daily timetable to follow, to ensure you get the maximum benefit from your food, iron tablets, supplements and nutrition alike. I have also provided a suggested three week menu plan with accompanying recipes.

In the following table I have identified foods that will *enable* the absorption of iron and should be eaten at the same time as iron rich foods, as well as foods that will *hinder* the absorption and should be avoided when eating your iron rich foods.

Iron Absorption Enhancers	Iron Absorption Inhibitors
Meat / Fish / Poultry	Polyphenols found in Red wine & chocolate
Vegetables: Broccoli, Brussels sprouts, potatoes, tomato juice, red, yellow, orange & green peppers	Tannins found in Tea, Coffee, Cocoa, Chocolate & Red wine. Avoid consuming at least 30 minutes, ideally 60 minutes, before and after any iron rich meal.
Fruits: Oranges, orange juice, kiwi fruit, strawberries, raspberries, blueberries, grapefruit & other fruits rich in vitamin C.	Spinach, chard, beet greens, parsley, oregano, sweet potato & rhubarb
	Whole grains
	Bran
	Antacid medications can also reduce the absorption of iron. Avoid consuming for 2 hours after an iron rich meal
	Food additive EDTA
	Phosphoric acid found in fizzy drinks

Iron Absorption Inhibitors should **not** be consumed with your meals as they will significantly reduce the amount of iron that you will absorb from your food. Ideally they should be avoided for a minimum of 60 minutes before and after consuming your meals. If you can leave it longer that would be even better. When I first started an Iron Enhancing Diet, I cut out all of the Iron Absorption Inhibitors (with the exception of coffee) for four weeks, in a bid to give my body the best chance of absorbing as much iron as possible.

Vitamin C from fruit and vegetables helps us to absorb iron whereas the tannins in tea, coffee, red wine and chocolate hinder it. In addition bran and high fibre cereals as well as spinach, chard, beet greens, sweet potato & rhubarb carry iron out of the digestive system, preventing absorption.

To further complicate matters, iron rich foods are sub-divided into "haem" and "non-haem" foods. "Haem" means it comes from animals and "non-haem" means it comes from vegetable based foods. "Haem" rich foods are much more readily absorbed than "non-haem" foods, where only approximately 50% 0f the food value is absorbed. In addition, the iron absorption-enhancing foods can also increase the absorption of non-haem iron rich foods. For example: if you are eating a non-haem rich meal of lentils or pulses, if they are prepared in a tomato sauce the available iron will be more readily absorbed because of the presence of vitamin C in the tomato sauce.

Complicated? Confused? Ready to give up before you have started? In anticipation of this, I have set out some guidelines when it comes to eating haem / non-haem food types, as well as a table of their iron values.

Your daily requirements for iron vary widely depending on your sex and age. Menstruating women will need almost double the daily iron requirements of men.

HOW MUCH IRON YOU REQUIRE EVERY DAY*			
	UK	**USA**	**Australia**
Children, 1-10 years	Unable to find government guidelines	10mg	Unable to find government guidelines
Teenage males	Unable to find government guidelines	12mg	Unable to find government guidelines
Adult males	8.9mg	10mg	8mg
Teenage & adult females	14.8mg	18mg	18mg
Pregnant women	14.8mg **	30mg	27mg Advised to seek medical advice before increasing intake
*Average RDA (Recommended Daily Allowance) for iron			

**The National Childbirth Trust Nutritionist, Rosemary Dodds states that although women are not losing iron through menstruation during pregnancy, they can become anaemic because of the body demanding more iron and vitamins, to supply both mother and baby.

Not only does the mother's blood supply have to increase to allow nutrients to pass to her baby, but the mother must also provide the iron required for the developing baby and placenta, from her own stores.

Therefore, I would have to query why in the UK, when we are statistically likely to be low in iron anyway, why pregnant women are not given any advice on increasing iron levels in their diet, as they are in both the USA and Australia.

Although in the UK the RDA for iron is lower than in both the USA and Australia, it will not do you any harm to consume more iron in your daily diet, unless you have been diagnosed with Haemochromatosis.

It may be advisable to keep below 30mg per day.

Haem Foods

This is the best way to get iron from your diet as Haem rich foods contain a much higher iron value and is more easily absorbed. Calves liver is one of the richest sources yet unfortunately a lot of people do not like eating liver. However, I do have one recipe that I suggest you try as it disguises the liver. All my family eat this bolognaise sauce despite none of them liking liver!

Warning: **Due to the high levels of Vitamin A contained in liver, pregnant women should not consume it as it may damage their baby.**

IRON-RICH FOODS		
Iron-Rich Food (HAEM)	**Iron Content (mg) (per 100g serving)**	**RDA % (Recommended Daily Allowance)**
RED MEAT		
Calf's liver	14.0	78%
Kidney	8.0	44%
Venison	7.8	43%
Heart	7.7	43%
Beef liver	5.7	32%
Beef	3.1	17%
Ox tongue	3.0	17%
Minced beef	2.2	12%
Lamb	2.2	12%
Veal	1.3	7%
Pork	0.9	5%
Gammon (boiled)	0.8	4%
Bacon (grilled or fried)	0.6	3%
POULTRY & GAME BIRDS		
Chicken liver	8.75	48%
Goose	5.0	28%
Pheasant	5.0	28%
Turkey (dark meat)	2.2	12%
Turkey (light meat)	1.4	8%
Chicken (dark meat)	1.4	8%
Chicken (light meat)	0.9	5%

IRON-RICH FOODS

Iron-Rich Food (HAEM)	Iron Content (mg) (per 100g serving)	RDA (Recommended Daily Allowance)	%
MISCELLANEOUS			
Black pudding	20.0	111%	
Faggots	8.3	46%	
Liver pate	7.3	40.5%	
Liver sausage	6.4	36%	
Haggis	4.8	27%	
Ham (lean)	1.4	8%	
Lunch Meat (2 slices)	0.9	5%	
Hot dog (1)	0.5	3%	
FRESH SEAFOOD			
Cockles	28	155%	
Oysters	8.0	44%	
Mussels	7.0	39%	
Whitebait	4.0	22%	
Clams	2.6	14%	
Prawns / shrimp	1.75	10%	
CANNED SEAFOOD			
Shrimps	4.5	27%	
Sardines	4.5	27%	
Anchovies	4.0	22%	
Pilchards	2.7	16%	
Tuna	1.3	7%	

Non-Haem Foods

Non-Haem foods can also be excellent sources of iron in your diet. However, they are not so readily absorbed by the body and you can lose up to 50% of their value as they pass through the digestive tract. Added to that, the Iron Absorption Inhibitors that I have already made reference to can further reduce their iron value, therefore it is important to make the most of the Iron Absorption Enhancers, particularly if you are vegetarian.

Meat proteins will act as an enhancer, as will any vegetables and fruit rich in Vitamin C. In addition, Jane Clarke (Nutritionalist who writes regularly for the national press) suggests taking a 100mg Vitamin C supplements with every meal to ensure maximum iron absorption is achieved.

IRON-RICH FOODS

Iron-Rich Food (NON-HAEM)	Iron Content (mg) (per 100g serving)	RDA % (Recommended Daily Allowance)
GRAINS & CEREALS		
Soya Flour	9.0	50%
Quinoa	7.9	44%
Amaranth	7.0	39%
Oats (porridge)	4.0	22%
Buckwheat Flour	3.9	22%
Barley	1.75	10%
Pasta	1.75	10%
Bagel	1.2	6%
Bread (1 slice, wholewheat)	1.0	5.5%
Bread (1 slice, white)	0.6	3%
BREAKFAST CEREALS		
Bran Flakes	20.0	111%
Ready Brek	13.0	73%
Special K	13.0	73%

Other brands of fortified breakfast cereals will contain between 4mg-8mg iron per 100g. Check the label.

PULSES (cooked weight)		
Lentils	3.5	19%
Soya Beans	3.0	17%
Cannellini Beans	2.9	16%
Red Kidney Beans	2.5	14%
Lima/Butter Beans	2.5	14%
Chick Peas	2.0	11%
Mixed beans	2.0	11%
VEGETABLES		
Jerusalem artichoke	2.2	12%
Watercress	2.2	12%
Potatoes (with skin)	2.2	12%
Tomato Paste	3.4	19%
Cabbage	1.5	8%
Pumpkin	1.5	8%
Butternut Squash	1.5	8%

IRON-RICH FOODS

Iron-Rich Food (NON-HAEM)	Iron Content (mg) (per 100g serving)	RDA % (Recommended Daily Allowance)
Spring Greens	1.4	8%
Peas	1.0	5.5%
Spirulina (1 tsp)	5.0	28%
Tomato Paste (1tbsp)	0.5	3%
NUTS		
Cashew	6.2	34%
Soyabean nuts	6.0	33%
Almonds	3.0	17%
Peanuts	3.0	17%
Pecans	2.8	15.5%
Walnuts	2.8	15.5%
Hazelnuts	2.2	12%
Pistachios	1.7	9%
SEEDS (per 2 tablespoon portion)		
Pumpkin	2.7	15%
Pine Nuts	1.8	10%
Sunflower	1.3	7%
Sesame	1.0	5.5%
Hemp	1.0	5.5%
DRIED FRUITS & JUICES		
Prune Juice (250ml)	3.0	17%
Figs	4.2	23%
Apricots	3.5	19%
Raisins	1.5	8%
Peaches	1.2	7%
HANDY MISCELLANEOUS		
1 tblsp molasses	3.5	19%
225ml Soya Milk	1.8	10%
1 egg	1.0	5.5%
1 egg yolk	0.7	4%
2 tblsp peanut butter	0.6	3%
100g Heinz Baked Beans	1.4	8%

HOW TO FOLLOW THE IRON RICH PLAN
The Influence of L-Lysine

L-Lysine is an essential amino acid which plays a key part in the growth of hair. It is also often found to be in very low levels in people suffering from low ferritin levels. Interestingly when a significant proportion of women on high iron and vitamin C intake failed to achieve the required ferritin levels, once L-Lysine supplements were added to the diet, most women went on to achieve their target ferritin levels and their hair volume subsequently increased. However, once the L-Lysine supplement was removed from the diet, hair shedding resumed several months later.

500mg L-Lysine Supplement

Whilst you are enhancing your iron levels, I would suggest you take one x 500mg L-Lysine tablet with your breakfast and then take a second one with your evening meal. This amino acid is known to enhance the body's ability to restore ferritin levels and is also a vital component in the building of healthy hair.

Please read the chapter on supplements to ensure you are getting the optimum nutrition to help your hair as much as possible.

100mg Vitamin C Supplement

As mentioned earlier, whilst you are boosting your iron levels it may be beneficial to take a Vitamin C tablet with each meal to enhance the iron absorption rates.

Menu Plan

I have laid out 28 days of suggested menus to ensure you are achieving a very good level of iron intake in your diet. By adding the spirulina each day and any of the suggested iron rich snacks, you will enhance your intake and hopefully boost your iron stores at a faster rate. I would also hope that at the end of four weeks, this style of eating will come more naturally to you.

The Menu Plan is designed to be a guide to assist you in trying out new recipes and incorporating iron rich foods into your diet. You will note that on many of the meals I leave the choice of vegetables, salads, accompaniments etc up to you to select. The Menu Plan will enable you to achieve your daily iron targets and also ensures that you will not be consuming Iron Absorption Inhibitors with iron rich food. It also leaves plenty of scope to make your own adjustments. If for example there is a food item that you do not like or cannot eat, then substitute it for something else of comparable iron levels.

The Menu Plan is designed to boost flagging iron stores over a short term period. The body can only absorb so much iron per day therefore it takes approximately 3 months to see a boost in your iron levels. Once you achieve an iron level with which you and your Doctor are happy, you will discontinue the iron tablets, supplements and spirulina.

PLEASE NOTE *that the menus are designed for adults and **not** children.*

A Typical Iron Rich Day

Here follows an example of how to achieve your iron requirements for one day

Breakfast (take 1 x 100mg vitamin C tablet with meal & 1 x 500mg L-Lysine tablet)

Food	Iron Content
40gm serving of iron fortified breakfast cereal such as Special K	5.2mg
125ml soya milk.	1.0mg
1glass fresh orange juice	
(acts as Vitamin C Iron Absorption Enhancer)	
total	**6.2mg**

Lunch (take 1 x 100mg vitamin C tablet with meal)

Food	Iron Content
Ham sandwich made with 2 slices of wholewheat bread,	2.7mg
1 thick slice of ham, mayo & a little salad	
1 Kiwi fruit (acts as vitamin C Iron Absorption Enhancer)	
total	**2.7mg**

Dinner (take 1 x 100mg vitamin C tablet with meal & 1 x 500mg L-Lysine tablet))

Food	Iron Content
Spaghetti bolognaise (using special iron enriched sauce)	7.25mg
150gms of bolognaise & 100gms dry weight of spaghetti	
Side salad of lettuce leaves & watercress with peppers,	1.5mg
tomatoes & cucumber in a homemade salad dressing &	
sprinkled with 1 tblsp toasted pumpkin seeds. (salad items	
act as vitamin C Iron Absorption Enhancers)	
total	**8.75mg**

Iron Rich Snacks

Food	Iron Content
50gms cashew nuts	3.1mg
50gms dried apricots	1.75mg
total	**4.85mg**

Day 1

Take any prescribed iron tablets with meals & ensure you space them out throughout the day

Breakfast (take 1 x 100mg vitamin C tablet with meal & 1 x 500mg L-Lysine tablet)

Food	Iron Content
40gm serving of iron fortified breakfast cereal such as Special K	5.2mg
125ml soya milk.	1.0mg
1 glass fresh orange juice	
(acts as Vitamin C Iron Absorption Enhancer)	
total	6.2mg

DO NOT DRINK TEA OR COFFEE FOR AT LEAST 1 HOUR

Mid-morning: *Mix aloe vera juice with mineral water or fruit juice, add 1 teaspoon of spirulina if you choose and use this drink to take 1 Magnesium B tablet.*

Lunch (take 1 x 100mg vitamin C tablet with meal)

Food	Iron Content
Ham sandwich made with 2 slices of wholewheat bread, 1 thick slice of ham, mayo & a little salad	2.7mg
1 Kiwi fruit (acts as vitamin C Iron Absorption Enhancer)	
total	2.7mg

DO NOT DRINK TEA OR COFFEE FOR AT LEAST 1 HOUR

Dinner (take 1 x 100mg vitamin C tablet with meal & 1 x 500mg L-Lysine tablet)

Food	Iron Content
Iron Boost Bolognaise (using special iron enriched sauce) (see chapter 10, recipes) & 100gms dry weight of spaghetti	7.25mg
Side salad of lettuce leaves & watercress with peppers, tomatoes & cucumber in a homemade salad dressing (see chapter 10, recipes) & sprinkled with 1 tblsp toasted pumpkin seeds. (salad items act as vitamin C Iron Absorption Enhancers)	1.5mg
total	8.75mg

DO NOT DRINK TEA OR COFFEE FOR AT LEAST 1 HOUR

Estimated Daily Iron Intake Total   17.65mg

Please note: Although the total consumption of iron is above the RDA of 14.8mg, remember that the absorption levels of non-haem sources is much lower than haem sources.

An above recommended intake of iron will not do you any harm in these quantities **UNLESS** you suffer from Haemochromatosis. The United States Food and Nutrition Board, "Dietary Reference Intakes: Minerals", states that 45mg is the upper daily limit of iron per day for adults.

On days where the menus fall below 14.8mg of iron per day, I have included a recommended snack chart. These snacks are interchangeable with snacks of equivalent iron value.

Day 2
Take any prescribed iron tablets with meals

Breakfast (take 1 x 100mg vitamin C tablet with meal & 1 x 500mg L-Lysine tablet)

Food	Iron Content
2 rashers of grilled bacon, 2 tomatoes, halved & grilled with 1 tablespoon dry fried pumpkin seeds. 1 glass fresh orange juice (acts as Vitamin C Iron Absorption Enhancer)	1.95mg
total	1.95mg

DO NOT DRINK TEA OR COFFEE FOR AT LEAST 1 HOUR

Mid-morning: *Mix aloe vera juice with mineral water or fruit juice, add 1 teaspoon of spirulina if you choose and use this drink to take 1 Magnesium B tablet.*

Lunch (take 1 x 100mg vitamin C tablet with meal)

Food	Iron Content
Grilled Venison burger in a wholemeal bap with ketchup, lettuce, sliced tomato & sliced gherkin 1 orange (acts as vitamin C Iron Absorption Enhancer)	10.0mg
total	10.0mg

DO NOT DRINK TEA OR COFFEE FOR AT LEAST 1 HOUR

Dinner (take 1 x 100mg vitamin C tablet with meal & 1 x 500mg L-Lysine tablet)

Food	Iron Content
Mussels steamed in apple juice with chilli, ginger, garlic & coriander with oven baked chips/fries & side salad of mixed lettuce leaves in a feta & hemp seed oil dressing. (see chapter 10, recipes)	8.0mg
total	8.0mg

DO NOT DRINK TEA OR COFFEE FOR AT LEAST 1 HOUR

Estimated Daily Iron Intake Total   19.95mg

Day 3
Take any prescribed iron tablets with meals

Breakfast (take 1 x 100mg vitamin C tablet with meal & 1 x 500mg L-Lysine tablet)

Food	Iron Content
Homemade granola (see chapter 10, recipes) with 125ml soya milk	9.7mg
1 glass fresh orange juice	
(acts as Vitamin C Iron Absorption Enhancer)	
total	9.7mg

DO NOT DRINK TEA OR COFFEE FOR AT LEAST 1 HOUR

Mid-morning: *Mix aloe vera juice with mineral water or fruit juice, add 1 teaspoon of spirulina if you choose and use this drink to take 1 Magnesium B tablet.*

Lunch (take 1 x 100mg vitamin C tablet with meal)

Food	Iron Content
Butternut squash & leek soup (see chapter 10, recipes)	3.0mg
sprinkled with hulled hemp seeds & served with either 2 slices	2.0mg
wholemeal bread or 1 wholemeal bap	
1 handful of grapes (acts as Vitamin C Iron Absorption Enhancer)	
total	5.0mg

DO NOT DRINK TEA OR COFFEE FOR AT LEAST 1 HOUR

Dinner (take 1 x 100mg vitamin C tablet with meal & 1 x 500mg L-Lysine tablet)

Food	Iron Content
Herb baked Chicken breast with puy lentils, peppers	1.2mg
& tomatoes | (see chapter 10, recipes)	3.5mg
total	4.7mg

DO NOT DRINK TEA OR COFFEE FOR AT LEAST 1 HOUR

Estimated Daily Iron Intake Total   **19.4mg**

Day 4
Take any prescribed iron tablets with meals

Breakfast (take 1 x 100mg vitamin C tablet with meal & 1 x 500mg L-Lysine tablet)

Food	Iron Content
½ grapefruit, poached egg on wholemeal toast	2.0mg
1 glass fresh orange juice	
(acts as Vitamin C Iron Absorption Enhancer)	
total	2.0mg

DO NOT DRINK TEA OR COFFEE FOR AT LEAST 1 HOUR

Mid-morning: *Mix aloe vera juice with mineral water or fruit juice, add 1 teaspoon of spirulina if you choose and use this drink to take 1 Magnesium B tablet.*

Lunch (take 1 x 100mg vitamin C tablet with meal)

Food	Iron Content
Quinoa salad with feta cheese & mixed seeds (see chapter 10, recipes)	9.7mg
1 handful of raspberries (acts as Vitamin C Iron Absorption Enhancer)	
total	9.7mg

DO NOT DRINK TEA OR COFFEE FOR AT LEAST 1 HOUR

Dinner (take 1 x 100mg vitamin C tablet with meal & 1 x 500mg L-Lysine tablet)

Food	Iron Content
Poached salmon (see chapter 10, recipes) with new potatoes (skin on),	0.6mg
carrots & green beans. Mix 1 tablespoon toasted pumpkin seeds &	2.2mg
sprinkle of lemon juice over the vegetables. Can serve with a dollop	0.5mg
of crème fraiche.	
total	3.3mg

DO NOT DRINK TEA OR COFFEE FOR AT LEAST 1 HOUR

Estimated Daily Iron Intake Total   15.0mg

Day 5
Take any prescribed iron tablets with meals

Breakfast (take 1 x 100mg vitamin C tablet with meal & 1 x 500mg L-Lysine tablet)

Food	Iron Content
40gm serving of iron fortified breakfast cereal such as Bran Flakes	8.0mg
125ml soya milk	1.0mg
1 glass fresh orange juice	
(acts as Vitamin C Iron Absorption Enhancer)	
total	9.0mg

DO NOT DRINK TEA OR COFFEE FOR AT LEAST 1 HOUR

Mid-morning: *Mix aloe vera juice with mineral water or fruit juice, add 1 teaspoon of spirulina if you choose and use this drink to take 1 Magnesium B tablet.*

Lunch (take 1 x 100mg vitamin C tablet with meal)

Food	Iron Content
100g Baked beans on 2 slices wholemeal toast	4.8mg
Mixed berries (acts as Vitamin C Iron Absorption Enhancer) with	0.65mg
2 tablespoons low fat Greek yoghurt, 1 teaspoon honey,	
1 tablespoon sunflower seeds	
total	5.45mg

DO NOT DRINK TEA OR COFFEE FOR AT LEAST 1 HOUR

Dinner (take 1 x 100mg vitamin C tablet with meal & 1 x 500mg L-Lysine tablet)

Food	Iron Content
Tuna pasta (see chapter 10, recipes) with large mixed salad of your	2.0mg
choice & homemade pumpkin seed salad dressing	
(see chapter 10, recipes)	
total	2.0mg

DO NOT DRINK TEA OR COFFEE FOR AT LEAST 1 HOUR

Estimated Daily Iron Intake Total   16.45mg

Day 6
Take any prescribed iron tablets with meals

Breakfast (take 1 x 100mg vitamin C tablet with meal & 1 x 500mg L-Lysine tablet)

Food	Iron Content
Buckwheat pancakes with ham & cheese (see chapter 10, recipes)	1.7mg
1 glass fresh orange juice	
(acts as Vitamin C Iron Absorption Enhancer)	
total	**1.7mg**

DO NOT DRINK TEA OR COFFEE FOR AT LEAST 1 HOUR

Mid-morning: *Mix aloe vera juice with mineral water or fruit juice, add 1 teaspoon of spirulina if you choose and use this drink to take 1 Magnesium B tablet.*

Lunch (take 1 x 100mg vitamin C tablet with meal)

Food	Iron Content
Large salad of your choice served with 50g cockles	14.0mg
(fresh or from a jar) and 1 slice wholemeal bread	1.0mg
1 kiwi fruit (acts as Vitamin C Iron Absorption Enhancer)	
total	**15.0mg**

DO NOT DRINK TEA OR COFFEE FOR AT LEAST 1 HOUR

Dinner (take 1 x 100mg vitamin C tablet with meal & 1 x 500mg L-Lysine tablet)

Food	Iron Content
Thai Chick Peas with cous cous (see chapter 10, recipes)	2.4mg
Side salad and dressing of your choice	
total	**2.4mg**

DO NOT DRINK TEA OR COFFEE FOR AT LEAST 1 HOUR

Estimated Daily Iron Intake Total   **19.1mg**

Day 7
Take any prescribed iron tablets with meals

Breakfast (take 1 x 100mg vitamin C tablet with meal & 1 x 500mg L-Lysine tablet)

Food	Iron Content
Porridge made with apple juice (see chapter 10, recipes) & hulled hemp seeds	1.4mg
1 glass fresh orange juice (acts as Vitamin C Iron Absorption Enhancer)	
total	**1.4mg**

DO NOT DRINK TEA OR COFFEE FOR AT LEAST 1 HOUR

Mid-morning: *Mix aloe vera juice with mineral water or fruit juice, add 1 teaspoon of spirulina if you choose and use this drink to take 1 Magnesium B tablet.*

Lunch (take 1 x 100mg vitamin C tablet with meal)

Food	Iron Content
Homemade liver pate (see chapter 10, recipes) with	3.65mg
wholemeal pitta bread & large side salad dressed with	1.0mg
feta & hemp salad dressing (see chapter 10, recipes)	
Blueberries (acts as Vitamin C Iron Absorption Enhancer) with	0.5mg
low fat Greek natural yoghurt, 1 teaspoon honey,	
1 tablespoon sesame seeds	
total	**5.15mg**

DO NOT DRINK TEA OR COFFEE FOR AT LEAST 1 HOUR

Dinner (take 1 x 100mg vitamin C tablet with meal & 1 x 500mg L-Lysine tablet)

Food	Iron Content
120gm Roast pork, roast potatoes (skin on), broccoli & cauliflower	1.35mg
with apple sauce	3.3mg
total	**4.65mg**

DO NOT DRINK TEA OR COFFEE FOR AT LEAST 1 HOUR

Estimated Daily Iron Intake Total	**11.2mg**

Additional Recommended Iron Rich Snacks
Select a couple of snacks that will take you over the daily goal of 15mg

Food	Iron Content
50g soya bean nuts	3mg
50g cashew nuts	3.1mg
2 tablespoons dry fried pumpkin seeds	2.7mg
50g dried apricots	1.75mg
50g cockles	14mg
Small can of sardines on 1 slice wholemeal toast	5.5mg
2 small bowl (50g) bran flakes	10mg
1 slice Iron Booster Bar (see chapter 10, Recipes)	2.5mg

Day 8
Take any prescribed iron tablets with meals

Breakfast (take 1 x 100mg vitamin C tablet with meal & 1 x 500mg L-Lysine tablet)

Food	Iron Content
2 eggs, scrambled, with 1-2 slices of wholemeal toast	4.0mg
1 glass fresh orange juice	
(acts as Vitamin C Iron Absorption Enhancer)	
total	4.0mg

DO NOT DRINK TEA OR COFFEE FOR AT LEAST 1 HOUR

Mid-morning: *Mix aloe vera juice with mineral water or fruit juice, add 1 teaspoon of spirulina if you choose and use this drink to take 1 Magnesium B tablet.*

Lunch (take 1 x 100mg vitamin C tablet with meal)

Food	Iron Content
Sandwich made with 100gms roast pork, mixed salad & chutney/ relish of your choice	2.9mg
1 apple (acts as Vitamin C Iron Absorption Enhancer)	
total	2.9mg

DO NOT DRINK TEA OR COFFEE FOR AT LEAST 1 HOUR

Dinner (take 1 x 100mg vitamin C tablet with meal & 1 x 500mg L-Lysine tablet)

Food	Iron Content
Beef chilli with kidney beans (see chapter 10, recipes).	5.05mg
Served with tacos, topped with finely chopped cucumber, tomatoes,	
spring onions, shredded lettuce, dollop of sour cream &/or guacamole	
total	5.05mg

DO NOT DRINK TEA OR COFFEE FOR AT LEAST 1 HOUR

Estimated Daily Iron Intake Total   11.95mg

Additional Recommended Iron Rich Snacks
Select a couple of snacks that will take you over the daily goal of 15mg

Food	Iron Content
50g soya bean nuts	3mg
50g cashew nuts	3.1mg
2 tablespoons dry fried pumpkin seeds	2.7mg
50g dried apricots	1.75mg
50g cockles	14mg
Small can of sardines on 1 slice wholemeal toast	5.5mg
2 small bowl (50g) bran flakes	10mg
1 slice Iron Booster Bar (see chapter 10, Recipes)	2.5mg

Day 9
Take any prescribed iron tablets with meals

Breakfast (take 1 x 100mg vitamin C tablet with meal & 1 x 500mg L-Lysine tablet)

Food	Iron Content
2 rashers of bacon with fresh grilled tomatoes, topped with	0.6mg
1 tablespoon dry fried or grilled pumpkin seeds	1.35mg
1 glass fresh orange juice	
(acts as Vitamin C Iron Absorption Enhancer)	
total	**1.95mg**

DO NOT DRINK TEA OR COFFEE FOR AT LEAST 1 HOUR
Mid-morning: *Mix aloe vera juice with mineral water or fruit juice, add 1 teaspoon of spirulina if you choose and use this drink to take 1 Magnesium B tablet.*

Lunch (take 1 x 100mg vitamin C tablet with meal)

Food	Iron Content
2 large tablespoons of humous (50gm) of your choice, served with	0.5mg
rice cakes and crudités of raw carrot, cucmber, red pepper & celery	
Raspberries (acts as Vitamin C Iron Absorption Enhancer) with low fat	0.5mg
Greek natural yoghurt, 1 teaspoon honey & sprinkled with 1 tablespoon	
sesame seeds	
total	**1.0mg**

DO NOT DRINK TEA OR COFFEE FOR AT LEAST 1 HOUR

Dinner (take 1 x 100mg vitamin C tablet with meal & 1 x 500mg L-Lysine tablet)

Food	Iron Content
Garlic fried seafood (see chapter 10, recipes) served on brown	10.0mg
basmati rice, with side salad of mixed leaves dressed with homemade	0.9mg
salad dressing (see chapter 10, recipes) & sprinkled with 1 tablespoon	
toasted pine kernals	
total	**10.9mg**

DO NOT DRINK TEA OR COFFEE FOR AT LEAST 1 HOUR

Estimated Daily Iron Intake Total	**13.85mg**

Additional Recommended Iron Rich Snacks
Select a couple of snacks that will take you over the daily goal of 15mg

Food	Iron Content
50g soya bean nuts	3mg
50g cashew nuts	3.1mg
2 tablespoons dry fried pumpkin seeds	2.7mg
50g dried apricots	1.75mg
50g cockles	14mg
Small can of sardines on 1 slice wholemeal toast	5.5mg
2 small bowl (50g) bran flakes	10mg
1 slice Iron Booster Bar (see chapter 10, Recipes)	2.5mg

Day 10
Take any prescribed iron tablets with meals

Breakfast (take 1 x 100mg vitamin C tablet with meal & 1 x 500mg L-Lysine tablet)

Food	Iron Content
Homemade granola (see chapter 10, recipes)	8.7mg
125ml soya milk	1.0mg
1 glass fresh orange juice	
(Vitamin C Iron Absorption Enhancer)	
total	9.7mg

DO NOT DRINK TEA OR COFFEE FOR AT LEAST 1 HOUR

Mid-morning: Mix aloe vera juice with mineral water or fruit juice, add 1 teaspoon of spirulina if you choose and use this drink to take 1 Magnesium B tablet.

Lunch (take 1 x 100mg vitamin C tablet with meal)

Food	Iron Content
Mediterranean Salad with feta cheese & mixed seeds	1.0mg
(see chapter 10, recipes)	
1 kiwi fruit (acts as Vitamin C Iron Absorption Enhancer)	
total	1.0mg

DO NOT DRINK TEA OR COFFEE FOR AT LEAST 1 HOUR

Dinner (take 1 x 100mg vitamin C tablet with meal & 1 x 500mg L-Lysine tablet)

Food	Iron Content
Stir fried turkey breast & mixed vegetables served with cracked wheat	2.1mg
(see chapter 10, recipes)	
total	2.1mg

DO NOT DRINK TEA OR COFFEE FOR AT LEAST 1 HOUR

Estimated Daily Iron Intake Total　　　　　　　　　　**12.8mg**

Additional Recommended Iron Rich Snacks
Select a couple of snacks that will take you over the daily goal of 15mg

Food	Iron Content
50g soya bean nuts	3mg
50g cashew nuts	3.1mg
2 tablespoons dry fried pumpkin seeds	2.7mg
50g dried apricots	1.75mg
50g cockles	14mg
Small can of sardines on 1 slice wholemeal toast	5.5mg
2 small bowl (50g) bran flakes	10mg
1 slice Iron Booster Bar (see chapter 10, Recipes)	2.5mg

Day 11
Take any prescribed iron tablets with meals

Breakfast (take 1 x 100mg vitamin C tablet with meal & 1 x 500mg L-Lysine tablet)

Food	Iron Content
40gm serving of iron fortified breakfast cereal such as Special K	5.2mg
125ml soya milk.	1.0mg
1 glass fresh orange juice	
(acts as Vitamin C Iron Absorption Enhancer)	
total	6.2mg

DO NOT DRINK TEA OR COFFEE FOR AT LEAST 1 HOUR

Mid-morning: Mix aloe vera juice with mineral water or fruit juice, add 1 teaspoon of spirulina if you choose and use this drink to take 1 Magnesium B tablet.

Lunch (take 1 x 100mg vitamin C tablet with meal)

Food	Iron Content
Venison burger either homemade, or bought from Sainsbury's or Marks & Spencer. Serve in a wholemeal bap with a side salad & salad dressing of your choice.	10.0mg
Handful of strawberries (acts as Vitamin C Iron Absorption Enhancer)	
total	1.00mg

DO NOT DRINK TEA OR COFFEE FOR AT LEAST 1 HOUR

Dinner (take 1 x 100mg vitamin C tablet with meal & 1 x 500mg L-Lysine tablet)

Food	Iron Content
Herby baked trout (see chapter 10, recipes), new potatoes (skin on), steamed mixed vegetables of your choice. ie: baby corn, mange tout, sugar snap peas, carrots. Water cress & crème fraiche sauce (see chapter 10, recipes)	3.3mg
0.5mg	
total	3.8mg

DO NOT DRINK TEA OR COFFEE FOR AT LEAST 1 HOUR

Estimated Daily Iron Intake Total   20.00mg

Day 12
Take any prescribed iron tablets with meals

Breakfast (take 1 x 100mg vitamin C tablet with meal & 1 x 500mg L-Lysine tablet)

Food	Iron Content
Porridge made with 125ml soya milk & seeds	3.1mg
(see chapter 10, recipes)	
1 glass fresh orange juice	
(acts as Vitamin C Iron Absorption Enhancer)	
total	3.1mg

DO NOT DRINK TEA OR COFFEE FOR AT LEAST 1 HOUR

Mid-morning: *Mix aloe vera juice with mineral water or fruit juice, add 1 teaspoon of spirulina if you choose and use this drink to take 1 Magnesium B tablet.*

Lunch (take 1 x 100mg vitamin C tablet with meal)

Food	Iron Content
150gm Jacket potato with 100g canned baked beans in tomato sauce	4.7mg
1 apple (acts as Vitamin C Iron Absorption Enhancer)	
total	4.7mg

DO NOT DRINK TEA OR COFFEE FOR AT LEAST 1 HOUR

Dinner (take 1 x 100mg vitamin C tablet with meal & 1 x 500mg L-Lysine tablet)

Food	Iron Content
Smoked oysters in tomato sauce on linguine (see chapter 10, recipes)	8.0mg
Side salad of your choice dressed with feta & hemp salad dressing	
(see chapter 10, recipes)	
total	8.0mg

DO NOT DRINK TEA OR COFFEE FOR AT LEAST 1 HOUR

Estimated Daily Iron Intake Total   15.8mg

Day 13
Take any prescribed iron tablets with meals

Breakfast (take 1 x 100mg vitamin C tablet with meal & 1 x 500mg L-Lysine tablet)

Food	Iron Content
2 rashers bacon, 1 fried egg, 2 grilled tomatoes sprinkled with	1.35mg
½ tablespoon sunflower seeds	
1 glass fresh orange juice	
(acts as Vitamin C Iron Absorption Enhancer)	
total	**1.35mg**

DO NOT DRINK TEA OR COFFEE FOR AT LEAST 1 HOUR

Mid-morning: *Mix aloe vera juice with mineral water or fruit juice, add 1 teaspoon of spirulina if you choose and use this drink to take 1 Magnesium B tablet.*

Lunch (take 1 x 100mg vitamin C tablet with meal)

Food	Iron Content
Soya bean & broad bean salad (see chapter 10, recipes) & 1 slice	0.5mg
wholemeal bread	1.0mg
Handful of raspberries(acts as Vitamin C Iron Absorption Enhancer)	0.65mg
with 2 tablespoons low fat greek yoghurt, 1 teaspoon honey,	
1 tablespoon sunflower seeds	
total	**2.15mg**

DO NOT DRINK TEA OR COFFEE FOR AT LEAST 1 HOUR

Dinner (take 1 x 100mg vitamin C tablet with meal & 1 x 500mg L-Lysine tablet)

Food	Iron Content
Iron Boost Bolognaise on 100gm (dry weight) cooked spaghetti	7.25mg
(see chapter 10, recipes)	
Side salad of lettuce leaves & watercress with peppers, tomatoes &	1.5mg
cucumber in a homemade salad dressing (see chapter 10, recipes) &	
sprinkled with 1 tablespoon toasted pumpkin seeds.	
(salad items act as vitamin C Iron Absorption Enhancers).	
total	**8.75mg**

DO NOT DRINK TEA OR COFFEE FOR AT LEAST 1 HOUR

Estimated Daily Iron Intake Total	**12.25mg**

Additional Recommended Iron Rich Snacks
Select a couple of snacks that will take you over the daily goal of 15mg

Food	Iron Content
50g soya bean nuts	3mg
50g cashew nuts	3.1mg
2 tablespoons dry fried pumpkin seeds	2.7mg
50g dried apricots	1.75mg
50g cockles	14mg
Small can of sardines on 1 slice wholemeal toast	5.5mg
2 small bowl (50g) bran flakes	10mg
1 slice Iron Booster Bar (see chapter 10, Recipes)	2.5mg

Day 14
Take any prescribed iron tablets with meals

Breakfast (take 1 x 100mg vitamin C tablet with meal & 1 x 500mg L-Lysine tablet)

Food	Iron Content
40gm serving of iron fortified breakfast cereal such as Special K	5.2mg
125ml soya milk.	1.0mg
1 glass fresh orange juice	
(acts as Vitamin C Iron Absorption Enhancer)	
total	6.2mg

DO NOT DRINK TEA OR COFFEE FOR AT LEAST 1 HOUR

Mid-morning: *Mix aloe vera juice with mineral water or fruit juice, add 1 teaspoon of spirulina if you choose and use this drink to take 1 Magnesium B tablet.*

Lunch (take 1 x 100mg vitamin C tablet with meal)

Food	Iron Content
Homemade liver pate (see chapter 10, recipes) with wholemeal pitta	4.65mg
bread & large side salad dressed with feta & hemp salad dressing	
(see chapter 10, recipes)	
1 kiwi fruit (acts as Vitamin C Iron Absorption Enhancer)	
total	4.65mg

DO NOT DRINK TEA OR COFFEE FOR AT LEAST 1 HOUR

Dinner (take 1 x 100mg vitamin C tablet with meal & 1 x 500mg L-Lysine tablet)

Food	Iron Content
150g Roast Chicken, roast potatoes (skin on), selection of 2-3 fresh	2.1mg
vegetables such as French beans, sugar snap peas, cauliflower,	3.3mg
broccoli etc.	
total	5.4mg

DO NOT DRINK TEA OR COFFEE FOR AT LEAST 1 HOUR

Estimated Daily Iron Intake Total   16.25mg

Day 15
Take any prescribed iron tablets with meals

Breakfast (take 1 x 100mg vitamin C tablet with meal & 1 x 500mg L-Lysine tablet)

Food	Iron Content
40gm serving of iron fortified breakfast cereal such as Special K	5.2mg
125ml soya milk.	1.0mg
1 glass fresh orange juice	
(acts as Vitamin C Iron Absorption Enhancer)	
total	6.2mg

DO NOT DRINK TEA OR COFFEE FOR AT LEAST 1 HOUR

Mid-morning: *Mix aloe vera juice with mineral water or fruit juice, add 1 teaspoon of spirulina if you choose and use this drink to take 1 Magnesium B tablet.*

Lunch (take 1 x 100mg vitamin C tablet with meal)

Food	Iron Content
1 Chicken Salad Sandwich. 2 slices wholemeal bread filled with	2.9mg
100g chicken, salad of your choice & mayo/chutney of your choice	
1 apple (acts as Vitamin C Iron Absorption Enhancer)	
total	2.9mg

DO NOT DRINK TEA OR COFFEE FOR AT LEAST 1 HOUR

Dinner (take 1 x 100mg vitamin C tablet with meal & 1 x 500mg L-Lysine tablet)

Food	Iron Content
Spicy bean cannelloni (see chapter 10, recipes)	2.0mg
Side salad & dressing of your choice	
total	2.0mg

DO NOT DRINK TEA OR COFFEE FOR AT LEAST 1 HOUR

Estimated Daily Iron Intake Total	**11.1mg**

Additional Recommended Iron Rich Snacks
Select a couple of snacks that will take you over the daily goal of 15mg

Food	Iron Content
50g soya bean nuts	3mg
50g cashew nuts	3.1mg
2 tablespoons dry fried pumpkin seeds	2.7mg
50g dried apricots	1.75mg
50g cockles	14mg
Small can of sardines on 1 slice wholemeal toast	5.5mg
2 small bowl (50g) bran flakes	10mg
1 slice Iron Booster Bar (see chapter 10, Recipes)	2.5mg

Day 16
Take any prescribed iron tablets with meals

Breakfast (take 1 x 100mg vitamin C tablet with meal & 1 x 500mg L-Lysine tablet)

Food	Iron Content
½ grapefruit, 2 poached eggs & 1 slice wholemeal toast	3.0mg
1 glass fresh orange juice	
(acts as Vitamin C Iron Absorption Enhancer)	
total	3.0mg

DO NOT DRINK TEA OR COFFEE FOR AT LEAST 1 HOUR

Mid-morning: *Mix aloe vera juice with mineral water or fruit juice, add 1 teaspoon of spirulina if you choose and use this drink to take 1 Magnesium B tablet.*

Lunch (take 1 x 100mg vitamin C tablet with meal)

Food	Iron Content
Mediterranean Feta Salad (see chapter 10, recipes) with 1 tablespoon	1.35mg
toasted pumpkin seeds	
1 handful grapes (acts as Vitamin C Iron Absorption Enhancer)	
total	1.35mg

DO NOT DRINK TEA OR COFFEE FOR AT LEAST 1 HOUR

Dinner (take 1 x 100mg vitamin C tablet with meal & 1 x 500mg L-Lysine tablet)

Food	Iron Content
200g shelled & cooked Mussels in tomato sauce on cracked wheat	14.0mg
(see chapter 10, recipes)	
Side salad & dressing of your choice	
total	14.0mg

DO NOT DRINK TEA OR COFFEE FOR AT LEAST 1 HOUR

Estimated Daily Iron Intake Total   18.35mg

Day 17
Take any prescribed iron tablets with meals

Breakfast (take 1 x 100mg vitamin C tablet with meal & 1 x 500mg L-Lysine tablet)

Food	Iron Content
Homemade granola (see chapter 10, recipes)	8.7mg
125ml soya milk	1.0mg
1 glass fresh orange juice	
(acts as Vitamin C Iron Absorption Enhancer)	
total	9.7mg

DO NOT DRINK TEA OR COFFEE FOR AT LEAST 1 HOUR

Mid-morning: *Mix aloe vera juice with mineral water or fruit juice, add 1 teaspoon of spirulina if you choose and use this drink to take 1 Magnesium B tablet.*

Lunch (take 1 x 100mg vitamin C tablet with meal)

Food	Iron Content
Watercress soup (see chapter 10, recipes)	2.2
1 wholemeal roll	1.5
1 apple (acts as Vitamin C Iron Absorption Enhancer)	
total	3.7mg

DO NOT DRINK TEA OR COFFEE FOR AT LEAST 1 HOUR

Dinner (take 1 x 100mg vitamin C tablet with meal & 1 x 500mg L-Lysine tablet)

Food	Iron Content
2 turkey burgers (see chapter 10, recipes) & noodle salad	3.8mg
(see chapter 10, recipes) sprinkled with 1 tablespoon toasted	
sesame seeds	
total	3.8mg

DO NOT DRINK TEA OR COFFEE FOR AT LEAST 1 HOUR

Estimated Daily Iron Intake Total 17.2mg

Day 18
Take any prescribed iron tablets with meals

Breakfast (take 1 x 100mg vitamin C tablet with meal & 1 x 500mg L-Lysine tablet)

Food	Iron Content
2 rashers bacon & 2 grilled tomatoes topped with 1 tablespoon dry fried pumpkin seeds	1.95mg
1 glass fresh orange juice (acts as Vitamin C Iron Absorption Enhancer)	
total	1.95mg

DO NOT DRINK TEA OR COFFEE FOR AT LEAST 1 HOUR

Mid-morning: *Mix aloe vera juice with mineral water or fruit juice, add 1 teaspoon of spirulina if you choose and use this drink to take 1 Magnesium B tablet.*

Lunch (take 1 x 100mg vitamin C tablet with meal)

Food	Iron Content
Mozzarella & green bean salad (see chapter 10, recipes)	1.5mg
1 slice wholemeal bread	1.0mg
1 orange (acts as Vitamin C Iron Absorption Enhancer)	
total	2.5mg

DO NOT DRINK TEA OR COFFEE FOR AT LEAST 1 HOUR

Dinner (take 1 x 100mg vitamin C tablet with meal & 1 x 500mg L-Lysine tablet)

Food	Iron Content
Grilled lamb chops served with cannellini beans & fennel (see chapter 10, recipes)	5.5mg
total	5.5mg

DO NOT DRINK TEA OR COFFEE FOR AT LEAST 1 HOUR

Estimated Daily Iron Intake Total	9.95mg

Additional Recommended Iron Rich Snacks
Select a couple of snacks that will take you over the daily goal of 15mg

Food	Iron Content
50g soya bean nuts	3mg
50g cashew nuts	3.1mg
2 tablespoons dry fried pumpkin seeds	2.7mg
50g dried apricots	1.75mg
50g cockles	14mg
Small can of sardines on 1 slice wholemeal toast	5.5mg
2 small bowl (50g) bran flakes	10mg
1 slice Iron Booster Bar (see chapter 10, Recipes)	2.5mg

Day 19
Take any prescribed iron tablets with meals

Breakfast (take 1 x 100mg vitamin C tablet with meal & 1 x 500mg L-Lysine tablet)

Food	Iron Content
Homemade granola (see chapter 10, recipes)	8.7mg
125ml soya milk	1.0mg
1 glass fresh orange juice	
(acts as Vitamin C Iron Absorption Enhancer)	
total	9.7mg

DO NOT DRINK TEA OR COFFEE FOR AT LEAST 1 HOUR

Mid-morning: *Mix aloe vera juice with mineral water or fruit juice, add 1 teaspoon of spirulina if you choose and use this drink to take 1 Magnesium B tablet.*

Lunch (take 1 x 100mg vitamin C tablet with meal)

Food	Iron Content
Homemade liver pate (see chapter 10, recipes), 2 slices wholemeal	3.65mg
toast with a side salad & salad dressing of your choice.	2.0mg
1 handful of berries (acts as Vitamin C Iron Absorption Enhancer)	
total	5.65mg

DO NOT DRINK TEA OR COFFEE FOR AT LEAST 1 HOUR

Dinner (take 1 x 100mg vitamin C tablet with meal & 1 x 500mg L-Lysine tablet)

Food	Iron Content
Grilled/fried tuna steak with a squeeze of lemon juice, puy lentils	3.5mg
(see chapter 10, recipes), steamed vegetables of your choice.	
total	3.5mg

DO NOT DRINK TEA OR COFFEE FOR AT LEAST 1 HOUR

Estimated Daily Iron Intake Total   19.05mg

Day 20
Take any prescribed iron tablets with meals

Breakfast (take 1 x 100mg vitamin C tablet with meal & 1 x 500mg L-Lysine tablet)

Food	Iron Content
½ grapefruit & a red omelette (see chapter 10, recipes)	2.0mg
1 glass fresh orange juice	
(acts as Vitamin C Iron Absorption Enhancer)	
total	2.0mg

DO NOT DRINK TEA OR COFFEE FOR AT LEAST 1 HOUR

Mid-morning: *Mix aloe vera juice with mineral water or fruit juice, add 1 teaspoon of spirulina if you choose and use this drink to take 1 Magnesium B tablet.*

Lunch (take 1 x 100mg vitamin C tablet with meal)

Food	Iron Content
100g Prawns with Cous Cous Salad (see chapter 10, recipes)	1.75mg
	0.5mg
1 pear (acts as Vitamin C Iron Absorption Enhancer)	
total	2.25mg

DO NOT DRINK TEA OR COFFEE FOR AT LEAST 1 HOUR

Dinner (take 1 x 100mg vitamin C tablet with meal & 1 x 500mg L-Lysine tablet)

Food	Iron Content
Chicken livers Stroganoff style on brown basmati rice	10.94mg
(see chapter 10, recipes) served with a side salad of your choice	
total	10.94mg

DO NOT DRINK TEA OR COFFEE FOR AT LEAST 1 HOUR

Estimated Daily Iron Intake Total   15.19mg

Day 21
Take any prescribed iron tablets with meals

Breakfast (take 1 x 100mg vitamin C tablet with meal & 1 x 500mg L-Lysine tablet)

Food	Iron Content
Porridge made with apple juice & seeds (see chapter 10, recipes)	1.4mg
1 glass fresh orange juice	
(acts as Vitamin C Iron Absorption Enhancer)	
total	1.4mg

DO NOT DRINK TEA OR COFFEE FOR AT LEAST 1 HOUR

Mid-morning: *Mix aloe vera juice with mineral water or fruit juice, add 1 teaspoon of spirulina if you choose and use this drink to take 1 Magnesium B tablet.*

Lunch (take 1 x 100mg vitamin C tablet with meal)

Food	Iron Content
100g baked beans on 2 slices wholemeal toast	1.4mg
	2.0mg
1 handful mixed berries (acts as Vitamin C Iron Absorption Enhancer)	
total	3.4mg

DO NOT DRINK TEA OR COFFEE FOR AT LEAST 1 HOUR

Dinner (take 1 x 100mg vitamin C tablet with meal & 1 x 500mg L-Lysine tablet)

Food	Iron Content
120g Roast beef, roast potatoes (skin on), vegetables &	3.72mg
accompaniments of your choice	3.3mg
total	7.02mg

DO NOT DRINK TEA OR COFFEE FOR AT LEAST 1 HOUR

Estimated Daily Iron Intake Total	**11.82mg**

Additional Recommended Iron Rich Snacks
Select a couple of snacks that will take you over the daily goal of 15mg

Food	Iron Content
50g soya bean nuts	3mg
50g cashew nuts	3.1mg
2 tablespoons dry fried pumpkin seeds	2.7mg
50g dried apricots	1.75mg
50g cockles	14mg
Small can of sardines on 1 slice wholemeal toast	5.5mg
2 small bowl (50g) bran flakes	10mg
1 slice Iron Booster Bar (see chapter 10, Recipes)	2.5mg

Day 22
Take any prescribed iron tablets with meals

Breakfast (take 1 x 100mg vitamin C tablet with meal & 1 x 500mg L-Lysine tablet)

Food	Iron Content
Buckwheat pancakes with ham & cheese (see chapter 10, recipes)	1.7mg
1 glass fresh orange juice	
(acts as Vitamin C Iron Absorption Enhancer)	
total	1.7mg

DO NOT DRINK TEA OR COFFEE FOR AT LEAST 1 HOUR

Mid-morning: *Mix aloe vera juice with mineral water or fruit juice, add 1 teaspoon of spirulina if you choose and use this drink to take 1 Magnesium B tablet.*

Lunch (take 1 x 100mg vitamin C tablet with meal)

Food	Iron Content
Beef salad sandwich made with 2 slices wholemeal bread,	3.1mg
100g sliced beef, salad of your choice & mayo or horseradish sauce	2.0mg
1 apple (acts as Vitamin C Iron Absorption Enhancer)	
total	5.1mg

DO NOT DRINK TEA OR COFFEE FOR AT LEAST 1 HOUR

Dinner (take 1 x 100mg vitamin C tablet with meal & 1 x 500mg L-Lysine tablet)

Food	Iron Content
Pan fried salmon fillet served with rice noodle salad	1.85mg
(see chapter 10, recipes) 1 tablespoon toasted pumpkin seeds	
total	1.85mg

DO NOT DRINK TEA OR COFFEE FOR AT LEAST 1 HOUR

Estimated Daily Iron Intake Total	**8.65mg**

Additional Recommended Iron Rich Snacks
Select a couple of snacks that will take you over the daily goal of 15mg

Food	Iron Content
50g soya bean nuts	3mg
50g cashew nuts	3.1mg
2 tablespoons dry fried pumpkin seeds	2.7mg
50g dried apricots	1.75mg
50g cockles	14mg
Small can of sardines on 1 slice wholemeal toast	5.5mg
2 small bowl (50g) bran flakes	10mg
1 slice Iron Booster Bar (see chapter 10, Recipes)	2.5mg

Day 23
Take any prescribed iron tablets with meals

Breakfast (take 1 x 100mg vitamin C tablet with meal & 1 x 500mg L-Lysine tablet)

Food	Iron Content
40gm serving of iron fortified breakfast cereal such as Special K	5.2mg
125ml soya milk.	1.0mg
1 glass fresh orange juice	
(acts as Vitamin C Iron Absorption Enhancer)	
total	6.2mg

DO NOT DRINK TEA OR COFFEE FOR AT LEAST 1 HOUR

Mid-morning: *Mix aloe vera juice with mineral water or fruit juice, add 1 teaspoon of spirulina if you choose and use this drink to take 1 Magnesium B tablet.*

Lunch (take 1 x 100mg vitamin C tablet with meal)

Food	Iron Content
110g Dry fried Haloumi cheese with large mixed salad & salad	0.9mg
dressing of your choice & 1 tablespoon of dry fried pine nut kernals	
1 orange (acts as Vitamin C Iron Absorption Enhancer)	
total	0.9mg

DO NOT DRINK TEA OR COFFEE FOR AT LEAST 1 HOUR

Dinner (take 1 x 100mg vitamin C tablet with meal & 1 x 500mg L-Lysine tablet)

Food	Iron Content
Venison Casserole (see chapter 10, recipes), boiled potatoes (skin on)	9.75mg
& green beans of your choice	3.3mg
total	13.05mg

DO NOT DRINK TEA OR COFFEE FOR AT LEAST 1 HOUR

Estimated Daily Iron Intake Total   20.15mg

Day 24
Take any prescribed iron tablets with meals

Breakfast (take 1 x 100mg vitamin C tablet with meal & 1 x 500mg L-Lysine tablet)

Food	Iron Content
2 eggs scrambled, served on 2 slices of wholemeal toast	4.0mg
1 glass fresh orange juice	
(acts as Vitamin C Iron Absorption Enhancer)	
total	4.0mg

DO NOT DRINK TEA OR COFFEE FOR AT LEAST 1 HOUR

Mid-morning: *Mix aloe vera juice with mineral water or fruit juice, add 1 teaspoon of spirulina if you choose and use this drink to take 1 Magnesium B tablet.*

Lunch (take 1 x 100mg vitamin C tablet with meal)

Food	Iron Content
Spicy lentil soup (see chapter 10, recipes), served with 1 wholemeal bap	3.5mg
	1.5mg
1 pear (acts as Vitamin C Iron Absorption Enhancer)	
total	5.0mg

DO NOT DRINK TEA OR COFFEE FOR AT LEAST 1 HOUR

Dinner (take 1 x 100mg vitamin C tablet with meal & 1 x 500mg L-Lysine tablet)

Food	Iron Content
Chicken & cashew nuts on brown basmati rice	1.23mg
(see chapter 10, recipes) Serve with a side salad of your choice	1.55mg
total	2.78mg

DO NOT DRINK TEA OR COFFEE FOR AT LEAST 1 HOUR

Estimated Daily Iron Intake Total	**11.78mg**

Additional Recommended Iron Rich Snacks
Select a couple of snacks that will take you over the daily goal of 15mg

Food	Iron Content
50g soya bean nuts	3mg
50g cashew nuts	3.1mg
2 tablespoons dry fried pumpkin seeds	2.7mg
50g dried apricots	1.75mg
50g cockles	14mg
Small can of sardines on 1 slice wholemeal toast	5.5mg
2 small bowl (50g) bran flakes	10mg
1 slice Iron Booster Bar (see chapter 10, Recipes)	2.5mg

Day 25
Take any prescribed iron tablets with meals

Breakfast (take 1 x 100mg vitamin C tablet with meal & 1 x 500mg L-Lysine tablet)

Food	Iron Content
2 rashers of bacon, 2 grilled tomatoes topped with	1.35mg
1 tablespoon dry fried pumpkin seeds	
1 glass fresh orange juice	
(acts as Vitamin C Iron Absorption Enhancer)	
total	1.35mg

DO NOT DRINK TEA OR COFFEE FOR AT LEAST 1 HOUR

Mid-morning: *Mix aloe vera juice with mineral water or fruit juice, add 1 teaspoon of spirulina if you choose and use this drink to take 1 Magnesium B tablet.*

Lunch (take 1 x 100mg vitamin C tablet with meal)

Food	Iron Content
Prawn salad sandwich made with 100g prawns, salad of your choice	1.75mg
and mayo on 2 slices wholemeal bread. Add lemon juice to	2.0mg
taste if required	
1 kiwi fruit (acts as Vitamin C Iron Absorption Enhancer)	
total	3.75mg

DO NOT DRINK TEA OR COFFEE FOR AT LEAST 1 HOUR

Dinner (take 1 x 100mg vitamin C tablet with meal & 1 x 500mg L-Lysine tablet)

Food	Iron Content
150gm Jacket potato with one serving of Iron Boost Bolognaise sauce	3.3mg
(see chapter 10, recipes) served with side salad of your choice	7.25mg
total	10.55mg

DO NOT DRINK TEA OR COFFEE FOR AT LEAST 1 HOUR

Estimated Daily Iron Intake Total   **15.65mg**

Day 26
Take any prescribed iron tablets with meals

Breakfast (take 1 x 100mg vitamin C tablet with meal & 1 x 500mg L-Lysine tablet)

Food	Iron Content
Grilled/fried fillet of trout with pumpkin seeds & grilled tomatoes	1.35mg
1 glass fresh orange juice	
(acts as Vitamin C Iron Absorption Enhancer)	
total	1.35mg

DO NOT DRINK TEA OR COFFEE FOR AT LEAST 1 HOUR

Mid-morning: Mix aloe vera juice with mineral water or fruit juice, add 1 teaspoon of spirulina if you choose and use this drink to take 1 Magnesium B tablet.

Lunch (take 1 x 100mg vitamin C tablet with meal)

Food	Iron Content
50gms cockles with puy lentil salad (see chapter 10, recipes)	14mg
	3.5mg
1 apple (acts as Vitamin C Iron Absorption Enhancer)	
total	17.5mg

DO NOT DRINK TEA OR COFFEE FOR AT LEAST 1 HOUR

Dinner (take 1 x 100mg vitamin C tablet with meal & 1 x 500mg L-Lysine tablet)

Food	Iron Content
Tuna bake (see chapter 10, recipes) with sweetcorn salad	2.0mg
(see chapter 10, recipes)	
total	2.0mg

DO NOT DRINK TEA OR COFFEE FOR AT LEAST 1 HOUR

Estimated Daily Iron Intake Total   20.85mg

Day 27
Take any prescribed iron tablets with meals

Breakfast (take 1 x 100mg vitamin C tablet with meal & 1 x 500mg L-Lysine tablet)

Food	Iron Content
40gm serving of iron fortified breakfast cereal such as Special K	5.2mg
125ml soya milk.	1.0mg
1 glass fresh orange juice	
(acts as Vitamin C Iron Absorption Enhancer)	
total	6.2mg

DO NOT DRINK TEA OR COFFEE FOR AT LEAST 1 HOUR

Mid-morning: *Mix aloe vera juice with mineral water or fruit juice, add 1 teaspoon of spirulina if you choose and use this drink to take 1 Magnesium B tablet.*

Lunch (take 1 x 100mg vitamin C tablet with meal)

Food	Iron Content
Stuffed peppers (see chapter 10, recipes). Can be eaten hot or cold.	0.6mg
Side salad & salad dressing of your choice	
Handful of berries (acts as Vitamin C Iron Absorption Enhancer)	
total	0.6mg

DO NOT DRINK TEA OR COFFEE FOR AT LEAST 1 HOUR

Dinner (take 1 x 100mg vitamin C tablet with meal & 1 x 500mg L-Lysine tablet)

Food	Iron Content
Thai Chick Peas on cracked wheat (see chapter 10, recipes) with a side salad of your choice	2.4mg
total	2.4mg

DO NOT DRINK TEA OR COFFEE FOR AT LEAST 1 HOUR

Estimated Daily Iron Intake Total   **9.2mg**

Additional Recommended Iron Rich Snacks
Select a couple of snacks that will take you over the daily goal of 15mg

Food	Iron Content
50g soya bean nuts	3mg
50g cashew nuts	3.1mg
2 tablespoons dry fried pumpkin seeds	2.7mg
50g dried apricots	1.75mg
50g cockles	14mg
Small can of sardines on 1 slice wholemeal toast	5.5mg
2 small bowl (50g) bran flakes	10mg
1 slice Iron Booster Bar (see chapter 10, Recipes)	2.5mg

Day 28
Take any prescribed iron tablets with meals

Breakfast (take 1 x 100mg vitamin C tablet with meal & 1 x 500mg L-Lysine tablet)

Food	Iron Content
Homemade granola	8.7mg
125ml soya milk	1.0mg
1 glass fresh orange juice	
(acts as Vitamin C Iron Absorption Enhancer)	
total	9.7mg

DO NOT DRINK TEA OR COFFEE FOR AT LEAST 1 HOUR

Mid-morning: *Mix aloe vera juice with mineral water or fruit juice, add 1 teaspoon of spirulina if you choose and use this drink to take 1 Magnesium B tablet.*

Lunch (take 1 x 100mg vitamin C tablet with meal)

Food	Iron Content
Homemade quesidas with goats cheese, red onions, tomatoes & basil	0.5mg
(see chapter 10, recipes) sprinkle with 1 tablespoon sesame seeds	
Raspberries (acts as Vitamin C Iron Absorption Enhancer) with low fat	0.5mg
Greek natural yoghurt, 1 teaspoon honey & sprinkled with 20gm	
chopped cashew nuts	
total	1.0mg

DO NOT DRINK TEA OR COFFEE FOR AT LEAST 1 HOUR

Dinner (take 1 x 100mg vitamin C tablet with meal & 1 x 500mg L-Lysine tablet)

Food	Iron Content
120g Roast Chicken, roast potatoes, vegetables & accompaniments	1.1mg
of your choice	3.3mg
total	4.4mg

DO NOT DRINK TEA OR COFFEE FOR AT LEAST 1 HOUR

Estimated Daily Iron Intake Total   15.1mg

CHAPTER 8

Is Candidiasis the cause of your hair loss?

I followed the supplement regime for three months and during that time, my hair grew back. However, after stopping the supplements, the hair loss resumed again within three months. Therefore, this indicated to me that the supplements were sufficient for my hair to grow, but without them I was not absorbing sufficient nutrition from my diet to maintain healthy hair. Hence my further studying the areas of low iron levels and Candidiasis influencing the body's ability to sustain hair.

As I have already explained in earlier chapters, for a long while I believed the cause of my hair loss could be attributed to low levels of iron in my body. This was qualified by the results of my serum ferritin tests and the medical practitioners I was seeing.

However, I later went on to question this as I was unable, after months of taking supplements and following an iron enhanced diet, to break the cycle of hair re-growing and subsequently falling out again. When my third serum ferritin test showed no increase in serum ferritin levels, I questioned if there was potentially a problem in my gut and its ability to absorb iron and other nutrients efficiently. It just did not make sense. I was consuming copious amounts, albeit in safe quantities of iron, but achieving no significant increase in my body's iron levels.

It was suggested that perhaps my body was building up iron stores, only to lose them each month during menstruation. The way to deal with this would be to go on the pill to either reduce menstrual flow, or to receive treatment to stop it completely. I was not happy with either of these scenarios. I came off of the pill a few years earlier due to problems experienced with it. The last thing I wanted was to throw my body into further turmoil with hormone treatment, particularly when I was convinced that it was more to do with my body's inability to absorb the iron. I said that I would think about it and went away and researched like crazy the absorption issues.

This was when I came across Candidiasis. Ironically I have been treated for this in the past when I suffered from ME. After eighteen months of ME symptoms, the treatment for Candidiasis cured me of those symptoms within six weeks. I was intrigued; could the same problem be presenting itself in a different way? Was it more than a coincidence that both the ME and hair loss had begun within two years of receiving very large doses of intravenous antibiotics? For the second time in my life I sought the advice/opinion of an Applied Kinesiologist and he confirmed that many people suffering from hair loss found Candidiasis to be the cause. Even better, once the Candidiasis was effectively treated, hair growth resumed and usually within a matter of weeks.

I was really excited at this news. Candidiasis is the overgrowth of unfriendly bacteria in the gut. There can be many triggers, including large doses of antibiotics killing off the friendly bacteria and allowing the candida to spread like wildfire through your system. Even better, the treatment is relatively simple. Follow a highly restrictive diet for a few weeks then re-populate your gut with friendly bacteria (in capsule form) and you should have killed off the problem.

The major drawback with this theory is in the United Kingdom, Candidiasis is not recognised by the medical profession, despite overwhelming research and documentation to support its existence. However, it is recognised in the USA, Canada and Australia and a Doctor in these countries will be able to offer advice which is currently unavailable here.

If you look up Candidiasis on the internet, there are lots of sites providing information and advice, but I could not find one definitive diet plan to follow. Taking all the advice I could find regarding what you should and should not eat, I devised my own plan which I then put into action. It was extremely difficult, particularly in the beginning as you are cutting out food types which are probably synonymous with everyday life. Giving up sugar for 6 weeks is not only difficult in itself, but also highly restrictive. Unless you prepare all of your meals from scratch, you will almost inevitably come across sugar in some shape or form throughout the course of your eating day!

However, I did manage to overcome this and this is laid out in the Anti-Candida Food Plan.

CHAPTER 9

The Anti-Candida Plan

The more I researched this area on how to eliminate candida from your body, the more confusing it became. If all advice was taken on board, you would end up on a highly restrictive diet which may not provide all of the daily nutritional requirements. In addition, it would probably be so difficult to stick to, that you would give up before gaining any benefit.

Depending on your current eating patterns, some people will find this plan easier than others to adapt to. Just keep in sight the motivation for doing it in the first place. ie: this may help you to re-grow your hair!

I am going to make the following suggestion. Follow the plan I have laid out for nine weeks if you can. I have made a three week menu plan, so just repeat it accordingly. If there is a meal that you do not like, substitute it for another one. Alternatively look at the recipes for the Iron Boost Plan as some of them will be compatible with the Anti-Candida Plan. All recipes identify which plan they are suitable for.

If you are really diligent, you may even be able to substitute a meal with a shop bought ready meal. However, due to the preservatives used in a lot of ready meals ie: sugar, they will be hard to come by.

At the moment Marks & Spencer do a delicious Tandoori Chicken Masala in 350g packs.

To try and make things as easy as possible whilst on the Anti –Candida Plan, I have written a notes column. For example: When you have a roast joint of meat, I will suggest that you put some of the cooked meat aside to be used in a meal in couple of days time. This is designed to save you time and some money.

Not all of the menus will give definitive quantities of food. For example: Certain meals will say "vegetables of your choice". You know how many vegetables you like to eat and which varieties. Just ensure that they are not on the 'What you *cannot* eat list'.

Where I have stated 'large salad' or 'side salad' of your choice, feel free to make up your own salads based on the ingredients you have to hand and if you so choose, select one of the salad dressings from the recipe section. *Please note:* you will have to make your own salad dressings as any ready made dressings I have seen contain vinegar or sugar or honey, which are all excluded on the Anti-Candida Plan.

Finally I would like to re-iterate that the plan detailed in this book is based on the menus I devised and followed for myself. If you are vegetarian, vegan or suffer from any food allergies or intolerances, you will probably require professional advice on devising a bespoke food plan to cater for your dietary needs.

Duration

For a six week period you will follow a "back to basics" diet. It will exclude a lot of foods that you may take for granted, but you will learn to become more creative at menu planning. If possible, try and extend it for a nine week period.

What you must remember is that the purpose of this diet is to **starve the candida in the gut**, to prevent it reproducing and spreading. One teaspoon of sugar, two weeks into the plan is enough to set you back to square one again, as you will have provided food for the candida. You must remember that the aim is to starve it out of your system.

For the first few days you may feel hungry. If this happens, snack on nuts, apples, seeds, permitted cheese or anything else on the permitted snack list.

Rules

You need to drink approximately 1½ - 2 litres of water a day.

Tea and coffee is permitted, but they must not have any added cow's milk or sugar

What you *cannot* eat

No fruit – with the exception of apples (limit to two a day) & lemon juice is permitted in cooking

No honey or syrup

No sugar – IN ANY FORM

Apart from the obvious, this will also include reading the labels on all food packaging. Anything that ends in "ose" is sugar ie: fructose, sucrose and lactose.

No artificial sweeteners – these will only serve to giving you sugar cravings. These can include Isomalt (also known as isomaltulose and palatinose). Sucralose (also known as E955) & sold as Splenda and Sucraplus. Sorbitol (E420) and all 'E' numbers E950-E969 which are categorised as sweeteners.

It is also worth noting that as 'E' numbers are being phased out on labelling, they are often replaced with their chemical name.

No dried fruit as this is high in sugar and can also have mould on it.

No yeast – as well as being in bakery products such as bread, crispbreads, crackers etc yeast is also found in **marmite, vinegar, soya sauce** and many fermented items– *read labels carefully.*

No smoked salmon

No Cow dairy products (unless it is guaranteed to be organic) – this includes milk and milk products, yoghurt, buttermilk, cream, butter and cheese. This is because non-organic cows are given antibiotics in their feed which can cause candida in the gut.

No Moulds or fungi – this covers **mushrooms, peanuts & certain cheeses**.

No high sugar vegetables – carrots, sweetcorn, peas and potatoes.

No alcohol – this converts to sugar and is also fermented (if you are absolutely desperate you can try gin or vodka, but beware of the mixers & remember it can potentially set you back).

No stock cubes – with the exception of Marigold Swiss Vegetable Boullion. Available in cubes or granules

No White Flours unless advised otherwise in recipes

No white rice – brown basmati rice is the most nutritious you can buy.

No White pasta – except for rice noodles

No ground pepper – has a higher likelihood of mould, but freshly milled pepper is fine.

No peanuts – has a high probability of mould even though this is invisible to the naked eye.

Eat three meals a day, plus snacks. If you are hungry, you must eat! You will probably feel very hungry for the first four to five days, particularly if refined carbohydrates and sugar features highly in your current diet. The hunger will gradually subside and after approximately two weeks, you may well find a substantial lack of appetite. However, you must still eat!

Try to have protein for breakfast. This will ensure you feel satisfied for longer.

What you *can* eat
Low carb vegetables, green vegetables, baby corn, cauliflower, aubergine, courgette etc
Sweet potato
Butternut squash
Brown rice – ideally basmati
Quinoa
Pulses – lentils, butter beans, kidney beans, cannellini beans, chick peas etc
All meats (ideally eat organic beef due to the presence of antibiotics in feed)
All fish
All shellfish
Game
Chicken
Salads
Hummus
Goats / sheeps cheese - ie: soft &/or hard goats cheese, haloumi cheese
Seeds – pumpkin, sunflower, pinenuts, sesame etc
Nuts – ensure they are fresh to avoid the risk of mould/fungal growth on them. For this reason avoid peanuts as they are the biggest culprit of exposure to mould which is almost invisible to the human eye.

Brown Bread – providing it is yeast free, sugar free. It would probably be best to substitute bread with rice cakes, certain brands of oatcakes and to make your own chapattis and tortillas. (recipes available in the plan).

Eggs – ideally use organic eggs as antibiotics are also added to the feed of non-organic chickens.

Remember to take your supplements. You may wish to take them with Aloe Vera juice, diluted in mineral water or apple juice. Aloe Vera contains many healing properties and can be soothing on your gut as you go through this process. However, it is optional. Health food shops sell Aloe Vera juice in a variety of different flavours and it is also packaged in various ways to address different ailments. You want to buy the plain, straight forward Aloe Vera juice with no extra additions or flavourings.

After six weeks you should be feeling the physical benefits of following the plan, although you probably will not see re-growth of hair yet. Do not be disheartened. You now need to reintroduce the "friendly" bacteria that we often hear on advertisements. The best way to do this is to purchase **Acidophilus Probiotics** in capsule form (see stockists list) and take it as per directions on the pack. The Probiotics should be stored in the fridge to preserve the shelf life.

We introduce the capsules at the six week point, when any Candida will have subsided significantly enough to allow the growth and colonisation of other bacteria in the gut. If you introduce it earlier you are potentially wasting your money, as the environment of the gut may not yet be able to support the growth of friendly bacteria.

Secondly we use capsules because they provide the optimum volume of bacteria. If you use the probiotic drinks and yoghurts available in the supermarkets, they not only contain sugar!!! But also have far lower numbers of bacteria. One capsule from the recommended brand claim *"Probably the UK's most potent probiotic - equivalent to 20 full pots of a leading supermarket's bio-yoghurt"*.

If after nine weeks of following the Anti-Candida food plan you see no improvement, then you should consider contacting an Applied Kinesiologist (please see supplier list for further details). They would be able to identify if you are particularly susceptible to certain food types (for example soya) and may need to follow a slightly different diet. You may need further assistance in identifying whether you require further supplementation in your diet, or testing to see if you are suffering from heavy metal toxicity (yet another potential candidate for causing hair loss).

Day	Meal	Notes
Saturday		
BREAKFAST	GO TO CHAPTER 10 FOR RECIPES	
	2 eggs, 1 rasher bacon, 2 grilled tomatoes	
SNACK	Small handful of Cashew nuts	
LUNCH	Lamb Bolognaise on wholewheat spaghetti & side salad	Keep half the bolognaise sauce to make Monday's chilli
SNACK	1 apple	
DINNER	Vegetable soup, mixed salad with cheese of your choice	Save half of the soup for lunch on Monday
SNACK	2 rice cakes & hummus	Use the recipe provided or buy from the supermarket.
Sunday		
BREAKFAST	Apple Porridge	
SNACK	1 apple	
LUNCH	Roast Pork, roast vegetables (peppers & onions) steamed green veg & homemade gravy	Keep some pork for lunch on Tuesday
SNACK	Toasted pumpkin seeds	
DINNER	Large mixed salad with grilled haloumi cheese, pinenuts & salad dressing	Grill 2-3 slices of haloumi cheese
SNACK	Homemade popcorn	
Monday		
BREAKFAST	Fillet of trout, lightly fried in rapeseed oil with a few pumpkin seeds and grilled tomatoes	
SNACK	2 rice cakes with creamy goats cheese	
LUNCH	Vegetable soup followed by bulgar wheat salad with prawns	Use soup reserved from Saturday
SNACK	1 apple	
DINNER	Chilli con carne on basmati rice with steamed vegetables or side salad	Keep some rice for lunch on Tuesday
SNACK	50g bag Clearspring Organic Japanese Rice Crackers	From Sainsbury's or Waitrose
Tuesday		
BREAKFAST	2 scrambled eggs with chopped spring onions & red pepper (raw or cooked) & oat cakes	Eat oat cakes if still hungry
SNACK	1 apple	
LUNCH	Stir fry the rice, pork & freshly chopped veg with sesame oil, garlic & lemon juice	
SNACK	Handful of nuts/seeds	
DINNER	salmon fillet fried in 1 teasp olive oil and served with a mixed salad & toasted pumpkin seeds	
SNACK	Crudites & goats cheese dip	Prepare muesli for tomorrow

Day	Meal	Notes
Wednesday	**GO TO CHAPTER 10 FOR RECIPES**	
BREAKFAST	Apple Museli	
SNACK	2 rice cakes & hummus	
LUNCH	Barley cous cous with 1 small can Princes mackerel in tomato sauce, heated and served on top & side salad	Check the ingredients of the mackerel sauce. Some have sugar in them. Barley cous cous sold in Sainsbury's. Best cooked in vegetable stock & forked through.
SNACK	1 apple	
DINNER	Puy lentils with oven roasted vegetables & Goats/feta cheese	
SNACK	Crudités / rice cakes & dip / hummus	
Thursday		
BREAKFAST	Grilled or fried Haloumi cheese with fresh sliced tomatoes, olive oil & dry fried pumpkin seeds	
SNACK	1 apple	
LUNCH	Butternut squash & leek soup. A large mixed salad with parmesan shavings on top	Save half of the soup for lunch on Saturday.
SNACK	Handful seeds / nuts	
DINNER	Turkey escalopes with green beans & pistachios & bulgar wheat	Cook double the quantity of bulgar wheat & reserve the extra portion for Friday.
SNACK	Feta & red onion dip with crudités and oatcakes	
Friday		
BREAKFAST	Apple porridge	
SNACK	Cashew nuts	
LUNCH	Bulgar wheat salad with mixed leaves & 1 slice of ham	
SNACK	Small portion of cheese & oat cakes	
DINNER	Stuffed peppers served with a side salad	
SNACK	Stewed apple (cook with a drop of apple juice) on rice cakes	

Day	Meal	Notes
Saturday	**GO TO CHAPTER 10 FOR RECIPES**	
BREAKFAST	Grilled bacon & tomatoes with 2 fried eggs	
SNACK	Goats cheese on oat cakes	
LUNCH	Butternut squash & leek soup. A large mixed salad with pine nuts & feta dressing	Use soup reserved from Thursday.
SNACK	1 apple	
DINNER	Freshly steamed mussels with home made chapatti & salad	
SNACK	Pistachio nuts	
Sunday		
BREAKFAST	Homemade buckwheat pancakes with ham, cheese & tomato	
SNACK	1 snack bag of Savour Bakes Oat Nibbles	
LUNCH	Roast chicken, oven roasted vegetables of your choice & homemade gravy	Keep some chicken for Tuesday
SNACK	1 apple	
DINNER	Rice noodle salad with soya beans	
SNACK	Bean dip on oat cakes	Keep some bean dip for Tuesday. Prepare muesli for tomorrow
Monday		
BREAKFAST	Apple muesli	
SNACK	Goats cheese dip with crudités	
LUNCH	Thai chick peas on barley cous cous	The chick peas can be prepared in advance & stored in the fridge.
SNACK	1 apple	
DINNER	Spicy turkey burger on chapatti with sticky red onions & mixed salad of your choice	Make a chapatti for tomorrow's lunch.
SNACK	Roasted spicy nuts	Prepare enough for tomorrow's snack.
Tuesday		
BREAKFAST	2 scrambled eggs with chopped spring onions & red pepper (raw or cooked) & oat cakes	Eat oat cakes if still hungry
SNACK	Spicy nuts	
LUNCH	Feta pesto salad with anchovies & olives	
SNACK	1 apple	
DINNER	Wheat free spaghetti with chicken sundried tomatoes, red onion & pine nuts	
SNACK	Bean dip with oat cakes	

Day	Meal		Notes
Wednesday		**GO TO CHAPTER 10 FOR RECIPES**	
	BREAKFAST	Apple porridge	
	SNACK	Roasted pumpkin seeds	
	LUNCH	Spicy lentil soup with a mixed side salad & feta cheese	Save half of the soup for lunch on Friday.
			Sold in supermarkets
	SNACK	Snack size sushi (do not use the soy sauce or pickled ginger)	
	DINNER	Chicken livers stroganoff style with vegetables of your choice	
	SNACK	1 apple	
Thursday			
	BREAKFAST	Haloumi cheese, tomatoes & pumpkin seeds fried in a little rapeseed or olive oil	
	SNACK	1 apple	
	LUNCH	1 small can of pilchards in tomato sauce, heated and served on barley cous cous with a side salad of your choice	Check there is no sugar in the ingredients on the can of pilchards
	SNACK	Roasted spicy nuts	
	DINNER	Peppered lamb steak with butter bean mash & vegetables of your choice	
	SNACK	Salsa & crudités	Shop bought salsa is fine as long as it does not contain sugar. (try Sainsbury's).
Friday			
	BREAKFAST	Grilled bacon with fried egg & tomatoes	
	SNACK	Hummus with rice cakes	
	LUNCH	Spicy lentil soup with goats cheese on rice cakes	Use soup reserved from Wednesday.
	SNACK	1 apple	
	DINNER	Pan fried salmon with rice noodle salad	Rice noodle salad is the same recipe but omit the soya beans.
	SNACK	Home made popcorn	

Day	Meal		Notes
Saturday			
BREAKFAST	**GO TO CHAPTER 10 FOR RECIPES**	Homemade buckwheat pancakes with ham, cheese & tomatoes	
SNACK		Hummus & crudités	
LUNCH		Quinoa salad with beans	
SNACK		1 apple	
DINNER		Chilli con carne with basmati rice & mixed leaves	Use half the quantity for the bolognaise recipe.
SNACK		1 snack bag of Savour Bakes Oat Nibbles	Soak muesli for tomorrow
Sunday			
BREAKFAST		Apple muesli	
SNACK		Homemade pop corn	
LUNCH		Roast lamb with home-made gravy & a selection of vegetables of your choice	
SNACK		1 apple	
DINNER		Pan fried fillet of trout, toasted pumpkin seeds with tomato & onion salad on rocket	
SNACK		Salsa. Crudités & rice cakes	
Monday			
BREAKFAST		Red omelette	
SNACK		Toasted pumpkin seeds	
LUNCH		Quesadilla with mozzarella, red onions, tomato & basil leaves	
SNACK		1 apple	
DINNER		Grilled or seared Tuna steak with butter beans & fennel and sugar snap peas	
SNACK		Homemade popcorn	
Tuesday			
BREAKFAST		Apple porridge	
SNACK		Snack size sushi (do not use the soya or pickled ginger)	
LUNCH		Feta salad & a chapatti	
SNACK		Pistachio nuts	
DINNER		Stuffed chicken breast with oven baked tomatoes & steamed green veg of your choice	
SNACK		1 apple	

Day	Meal		Notes
Wednesday	**GO TO CHAPTER 10 FOR RECIPES**		
	BREAKFAST	Grilled bacon with fried egg & tomatoes	
	SNACK	1 apple	
	LUNCH	Stuffed Cabbage Leaf Parcels with a side salad of your choice	
	SNACK	Goats cheese on rice cakes with cucumber	
	DINNER	Garlic fried seafood on basmati rice, with a side salad of your choice	
	SNACK	Hummus & crudités	
Thursday			
	BREAKFAST	Panfried trout, pumpkin seeds & tomatoes with a squeeze of lemon juice	
	SNACK	1 apple	
	LUNCH	Watercress soup with chapatti & mixed salad	Make an extra chapatti for Friday
	SNACK	Spicy nuts	
	DINNER	Spicy turkey burgers with butter bean mash & steamed vegetables of your choice	
	SNACK	Clearspring Organic Japanese Rice Crackers	
Friday			
	BREAKFAST	Apple porridge	
	SNACK	Roasted pumpkin seeds	
	LUNCH	Pancetta stir fry with broad beans & sugar snap peas serve with a chapatti	
	SNACK	1 apple	
	DINNER	Iron boost bolognaise on Wheat Free spaghetti with a side salad of your choice	
	SNACK	Homemade popcorn	

CHAPTER 10

Recipes for the Iron Rich Booster Plan & Anti-Candida Plan

Please note that each recipe will have a code next to it, indicating which of the plans it is suitable for. IR = Iron Rich Plan, AC = Anti-Candida Plan.

BREAKFASTS

Granola IR

30g porridge oats
1 tablespoon pumpkin seeds
1 tablespoon pine nuts
1 tablespoon sunflower seeds
1 tablespoon roughly chopped cashew nuts
2 dried figs, chopped
2 dried apricots, chopped
2 tablespoons honey
1 tablespoon sunflower oil (you can substitute sunflower for a different oil, except olive oil)
1 teaspoon ground cinnamon

1. Pre-heat the oven to 180c.

2. In a bowl mix the oats, seeds and chopped cashew nuts.

3. In a separate bowl, mix together the honey, oil and cinnamon. Then pour over the dry ingredients. Mix thoroughly with a spatula or spoon to ensure everything is coated.

4. Spread the mixture onto a baking tray and pop into the centre of the pre-heated oven for 25-30 minutes.

5. You may wish to stir the mixture every 10 minutes to ensure an even bake.

6. Once the granola is removed from the oven, cool and then stir in the chopped figs and apricots.

Note: why not increase the quantities to make a larger batch. The granola stores well in an air tight container.

Apple Porridge IR, AC

Serves 1

30g porridge oats
90ml apple juice
90ml water
5g coconut chips (optional)

Place the porridge oats, apple juice and water into a saucepan and bring to the boil. Simmer for 5-10 minutes until the oats are soft and have absorbed the liquid. Stir occasionally to prevent the oats from sticking.

Add the coconut chips at the end if you choose to use them.

Soya Porridge IR, AC

Serves 1

30g porridge oats
180ml soya milk
1 tablespoon of sesame seeds or seeds of your choice
Honey or maple syrup to taste (optional)

Place the porridge oats and soya milk into a saucepan and bring to the boil. Simmer for 5-10 minutes until the oats are soft and have absorbed the liquid. Stir occasionally to prevent the oats from sticking. Add the seeds and also honey or maple syrup to taste if required.

Apple Museli IR, AC

Serves 1

30g porridge oats
Apple juice
1 dessert spoon of chopped nuts
1 dessert spoon of mixed seeds (ie: sesame, sunflower, pumpkin)
1 apple, peeled & grated
Coconut chips (optional)
A pinch of freshly grated ginger (optional)

The night before put the porridge oats into a bowl and pour over sufficient apple juice to just cover the oats. If you are using the freshly grated ginger, add it at this stage. Cover and store in the fridge until the following morning. Add the remaining ingredients in the morning and serve.

Buckwheat Pancakes with ham, cheese & tomato
IR, AC

Serves 2

65g Buckwheat flour
Pinch of salt
1 egg
1 tablespoon of rapeseed or sunflower
oil + oil for cooking
100ml skimmed milk (preferably
organic)
2 slices of ham
50g grated cheese
2 medium tomatoes, sliced

1. Put the first 5 ingredients into a bowl and whisk with a hand or electric whisk until smooth. Ideally let the batter stand in a fridge for an hour before use.

2. Using an omelette pan or medium size frying pan, add 1 tablespoon of oil and heat gently, swirling the pan around until it is covered with oil. Any excess oil should be poured carefully into a heat proof bowl.

3. Test the temperature of the pan by adding a teaspoon of batter mix. If it sizzles immediately, the pan is ready.

4. Ladle enough batter into the pan to give a generous coating. Leave the pancake on the heat and after about a minute, it will have set and there will be no more runny batter. Flip it over to brown the other side which will take a few seconds. Transfer to a warm plate and add a slice of ham, some grated cheese and slices of tomato to one half of the pancake. You can add seasoning such as salt & pepper and chilli flakes at this stage. Flip the over half over to cover these ingredients. You can either serve at this stage, or if you prefer, return to the pan for about 30 seconds (turning half way through), to melt the cheese.

5. Repeat the above for the second pancake.

Red Omelette IR, AC

Serves 1

2 eggs
2 tablespoons milk
1 tablespoon rapeseed oil or olive oil
½ red onion peeled and chopped
½ red pepper, deseeded and chopped
1 medium tomato, seeds removed and chopped
Salt & pepper to season
½ teaspoon smoked paprika (optional)
Pinch of chilli flakes (optional)
Few sprigs of fresh coriander or parsley (optional)

1. In a bowl whisk the eggs with the milk and add seasoning to taste, including the smoked paprika and chilli flakes, if using.
2. Using an omelette pan or medium frying pan, heat the oil over a medium temperature, ensuring the pan is coated evenly with the oil.
3. When hot, add the onions and red pepper to the pan and cook gently until they have softened. Stir occasionally to prevent the ingredients sticking or burning.
4. Add the chopped tomatoes and cook for a further minute.
5. Pour in the whisked egg mix and cook until the eggs have set.
6. Garnish with the coriander or parsley and serve.

SOUPS

Butternut Squash & Leek Soup IR, AC

Serves 2

1 tablespoon olive oil
1 small onion, chopped
1 leek, washed and sliced
1 clove garlic either crushed or put through a garlic press
1 teaspoon cumin
1 teaspoon ground coriander
225g butternut squash, peeled, deseeded and chopped into cubes
425ml vegetable stock made with marigold stock cubes
Salt & pepper to season

1. Heat the oil in a large saucepan and add the onion, leek and garlic. Cook gently for 2-3 minutes.
2. Add the spices and seasoning and stir for another minute.
3. Add the squash and vegetable stock, then bring to the boil.
4. Cover and simmer for approximately 20 minutes or until the butternut squash is tender.
5. Remove from the heat, cool slightly and then purée the soup using either a hand blender or food processor.
6. The soup is now ready to serve.

Vegetable Soup IR, AC

Serves 2

1 tablespoon olive oil
1 small onion, chopped
225g of mixed vegetables of your choice ie: swede, sweet potato, parsnip.
425ml vegetable stock made with marigold stock cubes
Salt & pepper to season

1. Heat the oil in a large saucepan and add the onion. Cook gently for 2-3 minutes.
2. Add the vegetables and vegetable stock, then bring to the boil.
3. Cover and simmer for approximately 20 minutes or until the vegetables are tender.
4. Remove from the heat, cool slightly and then purée the soup using either a hand blender or food processor.
5. The soup is now ready to serve.

Spicy Lentil Soup IR, AC

Serves 2

1 tablespoon olive oil
1 small onion, chopped
Small piece of fresh ginger, peeled and finely grated (approximately 1 teaspoon)
1 teaspoon smoked paprika
Small pinch of chilli flakes
1 carrot, peeled and chopped
75g red lentils
450ml vegetable stock made with marigold stock cubes
Squeeze of lime juice
Salt & pepper to season
A small handful of fresh coriander leaves

1. Heat the olive oil in a large saucepan and fry the ginger and spices for a couple of minutes, stirring all the time.
2. Add the onion and carrot and cook for 5 minutes.
3. Add the lentils and stock.
4. Bring to the boil, cover and simmer for 15 minutes or until the lentils are tender.
5. Remove from the heat, cool slightly and then purée the soup using either a hand blender or food processor.
6. Add the lime juice and coriander and blend again.
7. The soup is now ready to serve.

Watercress Soup IR, AC

Serves 2

1 tablespoon olive oil
1 small onion, chopped
100g sweet potatoes
1 ½ sticks celery, chopped finely
100g watercress, roughly chopped
275ml vegetable stock made with marigold stock cubes
150ml coconut milk
Salt & pepper to season
Small sprigs of watercress to garnish

1. Heat the oil in a large saucepan and add the onion. Cook for 2-3 minutes.

2. Add the watercress, stock, coconut milk and seasoning, mix and bring to the boil.

3. Cover and simmer for approximately 15-20 minutes or until the vegetables are tender.

4. Remove from the heat, cool slightly and then purée the soup using either a hand blender or food processor.

5. The soup is now ready to serve.

SALADS

Crudités

Take a selection of raw vegetables, peel and deseed where necessary then chop into sticks. For example: cucumber, red/yellow/orange/green pepper, carrot, spring onion, celery. Baby corn and sugar snap peas also work well as crudités, but you may wish to blanch them for a few seconds in boiling water and then cool rapidly in cold water.

Mixed Salad – large salad or side salad

Use either one type of lettuce such as cos, romaine, baby gem or a selection of mixed leaves. I particularly like lambs leaf and baby spinach. This will be the base of your salad.

You can then experiment with a variety of raw vegetables to build up the body of your salad. For example: any of the above named items in the crudite section, try different types of tomatoes – usually the smaller tomatoes such as pomodorino have a sweeter more intense flavour.

Select a dressing from the dressings section and add to your salad just before serving.

You may wish to finish off your salad with a sprinkling of toasted nuts or seeds. Alternatively, or in addition you may wish to add shavings of parmesan cheese or hard goats cheese.

Bulgar Wheat Salad IR, AC

Serves 2–3

200g bulgar wheat
350ml vegetable stock – hot (made with Marigold stock cubes)
Juice of 1 lemon
50ml olive oil
1 teaspoon salt
½ teaspoon black pepper

Put all of the above ingredients in a bowl, stir then cover the bowl with cling film and leave for 1 hour.

½ cucumber, chopped
4 spring onions, chopped
Handful of cherry tomatoes, halved
Handful of fresh mint, chopped
Handful fresh parsley, chopped

Stir through the bulgar wheat and serve with a portion of protein such as cold pre-cooked chicken or some cooked prawns.

Barley Cous Cous Salad IR, AC

Serves 2

175g cous cous
225ml vegetable stock – boiling (made with Marigold stock cubes)
Juice of 1 lemon
1 tablespoon olive oil
¼ cucumber, chopped
4 spring onions, chopped
Handful of cherry tomatoes, halved
Handful of fresh mint, chopped
Handful fresh parsley, chopped
2 tablespoons pine kernals, dry fried until brown

1. Heat the olive oil in a medium – large saucepan. Add the couscous and stir until browned. This will take 2-3 minutes. Take off of the heat immediately.
2. Add the boiling vegetable stock and the lemon juice then cover immediately with a lid.
3. After 5 minutes "fluff" the couscous grains with a fork, then add the other ingredients and serve.

Rice Noodle Salad IR, AC

Serves 2

100g thin rice noodles

Splash of sesame oil

A handful of mange tout or sugar snap peas

1 red pepper, deseeded & thinly sliced

1 yellow or orange pepper, deseeded & thinly sliced

2 spring onions, trimmed & finely sliced

4 cherry tomatoes, halved

Handful of coriander leaves, chopped

1 400g can soya beans, drained & rinsed

Dressing

2 tbsp toasted sesame oil

1 shallot or ½ onion, peeled and finely diced

1 clove garlic, peeled and finely crushed

1 small red chilli, deseeded, finely chopped

2-3 tbsp lime juice, or more to taste

Splash of apple juice

1 tbsp toasted sesame seeds

1. Boil the kettle. Place the rice noodles in a heatproof bowl and pour on boiling water, ensuring that the noodles are fully covered. Cover the bowl with cling film and leave to stand for 5 minutes or until noodles are tender. Drain and toss with a splash of sesame oil to stop them sticking to each other.

2. In the meantime, blanch the mange tout in boiling water for 2 minutes until they are just tender but still bright green. Immediately run under cold water and drain well.

3. For the dressing, put all the ingredients into a bowl and whisk lightly to combine.

4. Put all of the ingredients into a large bowl. Pour over the dressing, toss well and serve.

Mediterranean Salad with Feta Cheese IR, AC

Serves 2

100g feta cheese, cubed
½ red onion, diced
2 beef tomatoes, sliced
¼ cucumber, cubed
Handful of fresh basil leaves, washed
6-8 olives
2 tablespoons dry fried/roasted pine nuts
3 tablespoons good quality olive oil
Juice of half lemon
Bed of lettuce leaves of your choice

1. Macerate the diced red onion by putting them in a bowl, add the olive oil and lemon juice and leave for at least 1 hour or overnight if possible.
2. Place the salad leaves on a serving dish and arrange the sliced tomatoes on top.
3. In a separate bowl gently mix together the onions with the olive oil and lemon juice, the cucumber and olives and pour over the tomatoes.
4. Sprinkle over the basil leaves and pine nuts and drizzle any remaining oil over the salad, then serve.

Mozzarella & Green Bean Salad IR, AC

Serves 2

100g cooked soya beans (canned or freshly cooked from either fresh or frozen)
100g blanched green beans or french beans, preferably fresh
125g pack of mozzarella pearls, drained (use balls or even chopped mozzarella if the pearls not available)
1 handful of small tomatoes, ie: cherry, pomodoro or even tomberries if you can get them
2 spring onions, washed and chopped
1 small red chilli, deseeded and finely chopped (optional)
1 handful of fresh basil, washed and chopped
2 tablespoons good quality olive oil
Juice of ½ lemon
Salt & pepper to taste

1. Mix the olive oil, lemon juice and salt & pepper together in a bowl.
2. Mix all of the other ingredients together in a serving bowl.
3. Pour over the dressing, add extra seasoning if required and serve.

Soya Bean & Broad Bean Salad IR

Serves 2

Mix all of the ingredients together in a bowl and serve.

100g cooked soya beans (canned or freshly cooked from either fresh or frozen)
100g cooked broad beans (canned or freshly cooked from either fresh or frozen)
1 small carrot, peeled and diced into small chunks
½ small red onion, finely chopped
1 small pepper, any colour, deseeded and finely chopped
1 portion of Vinaigrette dressing (see Dressings & Dips section)

Sweetcorn Salad IR

Serves 2

Mix all of the ingredients together in a bowl and serve.

198g can sweetcorn kernals, drained
2 medium tomatoes, roughly chopped
¼ large cucumber, deseeded and roughly chopped
2 spring onions, washed and sliced
2 tablespoons of a salad dressing of your choice (optional)

Feta Pesto Salad with Anchovies & Olives IR, AC

Serves 2

1 portion of Feta Pesto dressing
Anchovy fillets (I prefer the ones in
oil on the deli counters to the canned
ones)
A few olives of your choice
1 Cos Lettuce, washed and shredded

Put the prepared lettuce into a serving dish, pour over the dressing and toss the salad. Decorate with the anchovy fillets and olives.

Quinoa Salad with Beans IR, AC

Serves 2

150g quinoa, rinsed well under cold
water
300ml vegetable stock (use a
marigold boullion cube)
1 can mixed beans, drained and
rinsed
1 red pepper, diced
½ cucumber, deseeded and diced
1 carrot, peeled and shaved into
ribbons with a vegetable peeler
2 tablespoons pumpkin seeds, dry
fried in a frying pan until they are
browned and "popping"
1 portion Vinaigrette dressing (see
recipe in Dressing & Dips section)

1. In a saucepan, bring the stock to the boil. Then add the quinoa and leave to simmer for 10 minutes.
2. Pour the quinoa and stock into a heatproof bowl and cover with cling film. Set aside until the grains have absorbed the liquid.
3. Once the grains are ready, fluff them up by forking through with a fork.
4. Add the remaining ingredients and gently stir before serving.

DRESSINGS & DIPS

Linseed Oil has been used in these recipes for the optimum health benefits it offers. For further details please go to Chapter 19, Suppliers List.

Feta Pesto Salad Dressing IR, AC

Serves 2

1 clove garlic
1 handful fresh basil
25g feta cheese
50ml linseed oil (use cold pressed rapeseed oil or olive oil as an alternative)
100ml apple juice
4 small sundried tomatoes
Salt & pepper to season

Whizz all of the above ingredients together with a hand blender or in a food processor.

Vinaigrette Dressing IR, AC

Serves 2

75ml linseed oil (use cold pressed rapeseed oil or olive oil as an alternative)
Juice of ¼ lemon
1 clove of garlic, crushed
½ finely chopped shallot or ½ tablespoon finely chopped onion
½ teaspoon English mustard powder
40ml apple juice
¼ teaspoon dried mixed herbs
Sea salt & pepper to taste
Pinch of chilli flakes (optional)

Whizz all of the above ingredients together with a hand blender or in a food processor.
Note: This dressing is at its best when made in advance and left in the fridge for a few hours before using.
Please note: I have adapted Durwin Banks (High Barn Oils) recipe to make it comply with the Anti-Candida Plan.

Pumpkin Oil Dressing IR

Serves 2

4 tablespoons pumpkin seed oil
2 tablespoons wine or cider vinegar
1 clove crushed garlic
Salt & pepper to taste
Pinch of sugar (optional)

Whisk all of the above ingredients together with either a hand whisk or fork and serve.

Please note: pumpkin seed oil is very rich in iron & is full of flavour making it an ideal salad dressing on the Iron Boost Plan.

Goats Cheese Dip IR, AC

Serves 2

100g creamy goats cheese
25ml soya milk or goats milk
Pinch dried mixed herbs
Salt & pepper to season

Mix all the ingredients together and serve.

Bean Dip IR, AC

400g can of mixed beans, drained and rinsed
1 small red chilli, deseeded and chopped
1 stick celery, washed and chopped
1 shallot, finely chopped
1 tablespoon cold pressed rapeseed oil or olive oil
Salt & pepper to taste

Whizz all of the above ingredients together with a hand blender or in a food processor.

Red Pepper & Chickpea Dip IR, AC

2 red peppers, roasted, deseeded and chopped (from a jar if this is more convenient)
400g can chickpeas, drained and rinsed
4 tablespoons olive oil
1 clove garlic, crushed
Juice of ½ lemon
Small handful of fresh coriander, chopped
Salt & pepper to taste

Put all of the ingredients into a food processor or use a hand blender to blend to a smooth paste. Adjust seasoning to taste.

Remaining dip can be stored in a covered container in the fridge.

Hummus IR, AC

200g canned chick peas, drained and rinsed
100ml tahini
2 tablespoons olive oil
2 tablespoons lemon juice
2 cloves garlic, pressed
Salt to taste
Paprika to serve (optional)

1. Put all of the ingredients in a food processor and whizz until blended. Alternatively use a hand blender.
2. Adjust seasoning to taste. Sprinkle a little paprika over the top before serving.
3. Leftovers can be stored in a covered dish in the fridge.

Chicken Liver Pate IR, AC

Serves 2

1 tablespoon olive oil
1 small onion, chopped
1 clove garlic, crushed
350g chicken livers
3 tablespoons crème friache
2 tablespoons brandy
1 tablespoon tomato purée
1 handful chopped flat leaf parsley
Salt & pepper

1. Heat the olive oil in a non-stick saucepan. Add the onion and garlic and cook for approximately 5 minutes, until the onions are translucent. Stir occasionally to prevent burning.

2. Add the chicken livers and cook for a further 5 minutes until the livers are cooked. Stir regularly to prevent the livers from sticking.

3. Remove the pan from the heat and allow to cool slightly. Then add the crème friache, brandy, Tomato purée, parsley and season with the salt and pepper.

4. Put the mixture into a blender or food processor and blend until smooth. Transfer to a serving dish and cool.

5. Once cool, cover and store in a fridge until required.

MAIN MEALS

Chicken & Cashew Nuts on Brown Basmati Rice IR, AC

Serves 2

2 chicken breasts, cut into strips
100g mange tout
2 spring onions, sliced
2 handfuls baby spinach leaves
1 tablespoon sunflower oil
½ tablespoon sesame oil
1 tablespoon soya sauce 50g cashew nuts
100g dry weight brown rice

1. Put a saucepan of water on to boil for the rice. Add the rice to the boiling water and simmer for approximately 20 minutes.

2. Heat the sunflower oil and sesame oil in either a wok or large frying pan. When hot stir fry the chicken for 4-5 minutes and then add the mange tout, spring onions, cashew nuts and cook for a further 2 minutes. Finally add the spinach and stir fry until it has just wilted.

3. Rinse the rice with boiling water, place the rice in a serving dish, pour the chicken and cashew nuts on top and serve.

Herb Baked Chicken Breast with Puy Lentils IR, AC

Serves 2

2 chicken breasts – preferably with skin on
1 small onion, chopped
1 handful mixed fresh herbs of your choice such as parsley, tarragon, coriander, thyme or 2 teaspoons of dried mixed herbs
2 tablespoons cold pressed rapeseed oil or olive oil
2 cloves garlic, sliced into slivers
Juice of ½ lemon
Salt & pepper to season
125g Puy lentils cooked as per instructions or one pouch of microwavable Merchant Gourmet Puy Lentils

1. Pre-heat the oven to 180C & line a baking tray with tin foil, enough to make a parcel containing the chicken breasts.

2. With a sharp knife, make a few deep incisions into the top of the chicken breasts and then place on the tin foil.

3. Rub the oil all over the chicken breasts, then press some of the onion and slivers of garlic into the incisions. Sprinkle the remaining onion and garlic slivers over the chicken breasts.

4. Squeeze the lemon so the juice drizzles over the chicken, season with salt and pepper and lay the herbs on top. If you have chicken with skin on, loosen the skin by sliding your fingers underneath it and push some of the herbs under the skin.

5. Fold over the tin foil so that it makes a loose fitting parcel around the chicken breasts and bake on the middle shelf of the oven for approximately 20 minutes. The chicken is ready when a sharp knife is inserted into the meat and the juices run clear. If the juices are still pink or a little red, put back in the oven for a further 5 minutes and then test again.

6. Whilst the chicken is cooking prepare the puy lentils as per the cooking instructions. If you are cooking them I would suggest bringing the lentils to the boil in chicken stock and then simmer for 15-20 minutes until tender, then strain and serve.

7. Serve the chicken with the cooked lentils and either a selection of vegetables or salad of your choice.

Chicken & Spaghetti IR, AC

Serves 2

250g diced raw chicken – can be breast meat or thigh
1 red onion, peeled and chopped
8 Sundried tomatoes, reconstituted and chopped
50g pine nuts, dry fried and browned
2 tablespoons cold pressed rapeseed oil or olive oil
2 cloves garlic, pressed
Juice of ½ lemon
Small handful flat leaf parsley, chopped
Salt and pepper to season
200g whole wheat spaghetti

1. Put on a large pan of salted water to boil. When boiling add the spaghetti and cook for approximately 10 minutes. Stir occasionally to prevent the strands sticking together. Once the spaghetti is cooked, drain and rinse with boiling water from the kettle.

2. Meanwhile, in a large pan, heat the oil and add the diced chicken and chopped red onion. Stir continuously to prevent the meat from sticking. Do this until all of the chicken has cooked or browned on the outside.

3. Add the garlic and stir for another minute, then add the tomatoes, pine nuts and lemon juice. Keep stirring until the chicken is cooked.

4. Add the flat leaf parsley and a drop more oil if necessary. Season to taste then add the spaghetti and serve.

Stuffed Chicken Breasts IR, AC

Serves 2

2 chicken breasts
2 slices unsmoked bacon rashers
200g ricotta cheese
50g sun-dried tomatoes, reconstituted and chopped
Small handful of fresh basil leaves, torn
Salt and pepper to season

1. Preheat the oven to 190C.

2. Mix together the ricotta cheese, basil leaves, sun-dried tomatoes and season.

3. Make a horizontal incision across the chicken breasts and fill with the ricotta mixture.

4. Wrap each breast with a slice of bacon with the join underneath. You may wish to secure the breasts with a cocktail stick.

5. Place the chicken breasts on a baking tray and bake for 20-25 minutes or until the juices run clear.

6. Remove the cocktail sticks and serve with vegetables of your choice.

Chicken Livers Stroganoff Style IR, AC

Serves 2

200g – 250g fresh or defrosted
chicken livers
50ml organic milk or soya milk
2 tablespoons olive oil
1 small red onion, peeled and sliced
2 tablespoons organic crème friache
1 teaspoon English mustard powder,
mixed with a little water to make a
thick paste
1 tablespoon apple juice
1 tablespoon fresh parsley, chopped
Salt & pepper to season

1. Rinse the chicken livers, place in a bowl with the milk and leave to soak for 15-20 minutes. Drain and pat dry with kitchen paper.
2. Heat the oil in a frying pan. Add the onion and cook for a couple of minutes until softened.
3. Add the chicken livers and cook for a approximately one minute on each side.
4. Add the crème friache, English mustard, apple juice and parsley and simmer for approximately 5 minutes until the chicken livers are cooked. Season to taste before serving.

Lamb Bolognese Sauce IR, AC (for AC omit the carrot)

Serves 4 or 2 & reserve ½
for a chilli con carne

225g minced lamb
1 medium onion, finely chopped
1 large carrot, finely grated
1 dessertspoon of rapeseed or olive
oil
2 cloves of garlic either pressed or
finely chopped
2 teaspoons of dried mixed herbs
2 tablespoons tomato purée
1 can (400g) plum tomatoes
150ml of stock, water or apple juice
200g dry weight wholewheat
spaghetti

1. Heat a frying pan and add the oil, mince, chopped onion and grated carrot. Keep stirring breaking up any large lumps of meat, until all of the mince is browned.
2. Stir in the garlic and the herbs and cook for 2 minutes.
3. Stir in the tomato purée, tomatoes, 150ml of liquid of your choice and season well.
4. Simmer gently for 40-50 minutes until thick, stirring occasionally to prevent sticking to the bottom of the pan.
5. Whilst the Bolognese is cooking, bring a large pan of water to the boil for the spaghetti. Add to the boiling water for 10 minutes, stirring occasionally to prevent it sticking together.
6. Once the spaghetti is cooked, rinse it with plenty of freshly boiled water from a kettle. Once again, this helps to prevent all the strands sticking together.
7. Prepare a side salad whilst the Bolognese and spaghetti is cooking.

Iron Boost Bolognaise IR, AC (for AC omit the carrot)

Serves 2

125g minced lamb
100g lambs liver
200ml-250ml organic milk
1 medium onion, finely chopped
1 large carrot, finely grated
1 dessertspoon of rapeseed or olive oil
2 cloves of garlic either pressed or finely chopped
2 teaspoons of dried mixed herbs
2 tablespoons tomato purée
1 can (400g) plum tomatoes
150ml of stock, water or apple juice
200g dry weight wholewheat spaghetti

1. Soak the lambs liver in a bowl of organic milk for 1 hour in the fridge. Pat dry with kitchen paper then purée in a food processor or with a hand blender.

2. Heat a frying pan and add the oil, mince, puréed liver, chopped onion and grated carrot. Keep stirring breaking up any large lumps of meat, until all of the meat is browned.

3. Stir in the garlic and the herbs and cook for 2 minutes.

4. Stir in the tomato purée, tomatoes, 150ml of liquid of your choice and season well.

5. Simmer gently for 40-50 minutes until thick, stirring occasionally to prevent sticking to the bottom of the pan.

6. Whilst the Bolognese is cooking, bring a large pan of water to the boil for the spaghetti. Add to the boiling water for 10 minutes, stirring occasionally to prevent it sticking together.

7. Once the spaghetti is cooked, rinse it with plenty of freshly boiled water from a kettle. Once again, this helps to prevent all the strands sticking together.

8. Prepare a side salad whilst the Bolognese and spaghetti is cooking.

Lamb Chilli Con Carne IR, AC

Serves 2

Use half the quantity of the prepared Lamb Bolognese Sauce
1 small can kidney beans, drained and rinsed
1-2 teaspoons of chilli flakes, or 2 teaspoons mild chilli powder or of 1 teaspoon hot chilli powder
150g basmati rice — if you want to prepare extra for another meal, double the quantity. Remember to chill the extra rice with cold water & store in the fridge.

1. Put the Bolognese sauce into a pan and add the chilli and kidney beans. Reheat at a moderate temperature. Stir occasionally to prevent sticking. You may wish to add some extra liquid if the sauce is very thick.
2. Ensure that the sauce is piping hot before serving. Ideally let it simmer for 10-15 minutes to reach a temperature of 75c or above.
3. In the meantime cook your basmati rice in boiling water for approximately 10 minutes.
4. Prepare a side salad or steamed vegetables whilst the chilli and rice is cooking.

Peppered Lamb Steaks IR, AC

Serves 2

2 lamb steaks, approximately 140g each
1 tablespoon cold pressed rapeseed oil or olive oil
Freshly milled black pepper & sea salt

1. Liberally cover the lamb steaks in freshly ground black pepper and sprinkle on a little sea salt.
2. Heat the oil in a frying pan until very hot.
3. Cook the lamb steaks for approximately 3 minutes on each side if you like them pink or longer to suit your taste.
4. Serve with minted butter bean mash and steamed green vegetables.

Stir Fry Pork & Vegetables IR

Serves 2

200g cooked pork, diced
1 onion, peeled and sliced
100g sugar snap peas or mange tout
100g baby corn
1 carrot, peeled and cut into ribbons
with a vegetable peeler
225g-250g cooked rice (preferably
basmati)
1-2 tablespoons sesame oil
50ml apple juice
1 clove garlic, pressed
½ thumb size portion of fresh
ginger, peeled and grated
Juice of ½ lemon
Handful flat leaf parsley, chopped
Salt & pepper to season

1. eat the oil in a large pan and stir fry the vegetables for a couple of minutes.
2. Add the garlic, pork, cooked rice and apple juice and continue to cook for a few minutes until heated through.
3. Add the lemon juice, flat leaf parsley and season to taste.

Turkey Escalopes IR, AC

Serves 2

2 turkey escalopes
4 tablespoons Buckwheat flour
1 egg, beaten
50g porridge oats
1 teaspoon mustard powder
Salt and pepper
Pinch of chilli flakes (optional)
2 tablespoons vegetable oil

1. Put the buckwheat flour into a bowl and stir though the mustard powder.
2. Put a beaten egg into a bowl.
3. Put the porridge oats in a bowl and season with salt & pepper and chilli flakes.
4. Coat the escalopes in flour, shaking off the excess, dip in the egg and finally the porridge oats.
5. Heat the vegetable oil in a large frying pan and fry for 5 minutes on each side or until the juices run clear when cut with a knife.
6. Serve with green beans & pistachios.

Stir Fry Turkey on a bed of Bulgur Wheat IR, AC

Serves 2

200g turkey breast, cut into strips
1 red onion, sliced
1 large carrot, peeled and cut into
ribbons with a vegetable peeler
1 pepper, any colour, deseeded and
sliced
1 tablespoon pine nuts
1 handful coriander, chopped
1 clove garlic, crushed
1 ½ tablespoons sunflower oil
½ tablespoon sesame oil
Juice ½ lemon
Salt and pepper to season
100g bulgur wheat
100ml hot chicken stock (can be
made from a stock cube)

1. Put the bulgur wheat, lemon juice, sesame oil in a heat proof bowl and pour over the hot chicken stock. Cover with cling film and set aside for 1 hour.

2. In a wok or large frying pan heat the sunflower oil. When the oil is hot add the turkey breast, sliced red onion and stir fry for approximately 5 minutes. Then add the crushed garlic, carrot ribbons, sliced pepper and pine nuts and continue to stir fry for a couple more minutes.

3. Finally, add the coriander and season with salt and pepper to taste.

4. Before serving, you may wish to microwave the bulgur wheat for 1 minute to warm it through.

Spicy Turkey Burger IR, AC

Serves 2

250g lean turkey mince
½ apple, peeled & coarsely grated
2 spring onions, finely sliced
Small piece of fresh root ginger,
peeled & finely chopped or grated
Handful of fresh coriander, roughly
chopped
2 teaspoons garam masala
Salt & pepper to season
2 tablespoons gluten free flour. Soya
flour, rice flour or gram flour works
just as well
A drop of cold pressed rapeseed oil or
sunflower to shallow fry

1. With the exception of the flour and the oil for frying, put all of the ingredients into a bowl and mix together.

2. Sprinkle the flour onto a dinner plate.

3. Divide the mixture into 4 equal portions and then, using your hands, shape each portion into a burger shaped patty. Put them onto the floured plate and then turn to ensure each patty has a light, yet even coating of flour.

4. Heat the oil in a frying pan. Preferably use a heavy based, non-stick pan to ensure even cooking & the need for very little cooking oil.

5. Cook the patties for 3-4 minutes on each side. When you think they are cooked, cut into the centre to make sure they are not still pink.

6. Sticky red onions go really well with these spicy turkey burgers.

Venison Casserole IR

Serves 2

½ tablespoon olive oil
½ rounded tablespoon butter
1 medium onion, diced
2 clove garlic, crushed
2 rashers bacon, smoked or
unsmoked, chopped
250g mushrooms, sliced
1,000g – 1,250g boneless venison,
diced
50g cornflour
¼ bottle red wine
1 beef stock cube dissolved in 200ml
boiling water
2 tablespoons redcurrant jelly
Salt and pepper to season

1. Preheat the oven to 150c/330f.

2. In an ovenproof dish, heat the oil and butter on top of the hob. Add the onions and cook until soft and translucent.

3. Add the garlic, bacon and mushrooms and cook for a further minute.

4. In a separate frying pan, brown the venison a large spoonful at a time (if you cook too much meat at any one time, it will not brown). Once browned, add the meat to the casserole dish.

5. Add the red wine, stock, redcurrant jelly and season with the salt and pepper.

6. Bring to the boil on the hob. Once boiling, give the casserole a stir, then place on the lid. Cook in the middle of the oven for approximately 90 minutes.

7. Remove the casserole from the oven and put onto the hob.

8. Mix the cornflour with 2 tablespoons water into a smooth paste. Add a little at a time to the casserole, stirring frequently. The cornflour will make the gravy thicken. Leave to simmer for 5 minutes before serving.

Stuffed Cabbage Leaves IR, AC

Serves 2

4 large cabbage leaves
1 tablespoon olive oil
1 onion, peeled and chopped
250g turkey mince
1 red chilli, deseeded and chopped
1 carrot, peeled and grated
½ thumb size piece of fresh ginger,
peeled and grated
1 teaspoon smoked paprika
50g creamy goats cheese
50g cooked basmati rice
50ml apple juice
Salt and pepper to taste

1. Preheat the oven to 180c.

2. Cook the cabbage leaves for 2 minutes in a large pan of boiling water.

3. Remove the stalky section of the cabbage leaves with a sharp knife

4. Heat the olive oil in a pan and add the turkey mince, chopped onion, red chilli, grated carrot, ginger and parika. Cook until the meat is no longer pink, stirring occasionally to prevent sticking. Add the apple juice and simmer for another 5 minutes.

5. Take the pan off of the heat and add the creamy goats cheese, basmati rice and season to taste.

6. Pile the mixture up in the centre of the cabbage leaves. Carefully wrap the leaves around the mixture and if need be, secure with cocktail sticks.

7. Place the cabbage leaf parcels in a lightly oiled dish and add a drop of apple juice. Cover with tin foil and bake at 180c for 30 minutes. Serve with a side salad of your choice.

Stuffed Peppers IR, AC

Serves 2

2 Large peppers, the colour of your choice

225-250g cooked rice (preferably basmati)

4 spring onions, chopped

4 sundried tomatoes, chopped

1 tablespoon sesame seeds

1 tablespoon sunflower seeds

Juice of ½ lemon

2 tablespoons olive oil

1 teaspoon cumin

1 teaspoon paprika (smoked if you have it)

1 teaspoon chilli flakes (optional)

Salt & pepper to season

Tomato passatta to bind the mixture

2 tablespoons grated parmesan cheese

1. Preheat the oven to 180c.

2. Cut the peppers in half, deseed and remove the white pith.

3. With the exception of the passatta and parmesan cheese, mix all of the ingredients together in a bowl.

4. Add enough passatta to make the mixture bind together, but not be too runny.

5. Taste and adjust seasoning if necessary.

6. Carefully spoon the mixture into the 4 halves of pepper.

7. Sprinkle the grated parmesan on top and place the peppers on a baking sheet.

8. Bake for approximately 30 minutes. The peppers should be soft, the cheese golden on top and the rice mixture should be piping hot.

9. Serve with a side salad of your choice.

Steamed Mussels IR, AC

Serves 2

1 net of live mussels to serve 2 people (check at the fish counter in supermarkets)
1 red onion, peeled and finely chopped
1 red chilli, deseeded and finely chopped
1 thumb size piece of fresh ginger, peeled and finely chopped
1 clove garlic, pressed
1 tablespoon olive oil
Small handful of fresh coriander
200ml apple juice
Freshly ground pepper

1. Prepare the mussels for cooking. Firstly check that they are all tightly closed. If not, tap them with the edge of a knife. If the mussel closes it is alive, if not it is dead and therefore must be discarded. DO NOT cook dead mussels. Give them a scrub under cold running water, removing any barnacles with a knife and the hairy beard part.

2. Select a large saucepan with a tight fitting lid. Heat the oil in the saucepan and add the onion and chilli. Stir until softened, then add the garlic and ginger and stir for another minute.

3. Add the apple juice, coriander and pepper and allow the stock to come to the boil.

4. As soon as the stock is boiling, add the mussels and put on the lid immediately. They will be ready after approximately 5 minutes, depending on the size of the mussels. Take the lid off the saucepan and the mussels should be open. Discard any mussels that have not opened during cooking.

5. Serve in bowls accompanied with a chapatti and salad of your choice.

Mussels in Tomato Sauce on Cracked Wheat IR, AC

Serves 2

*200g fresh cooked mussels, no shells
(fish section of supermarkets)
400g can tomatoes (preferably
chopped or you can do this yourself)
2 tablespoons tomato purée
1 medium onion, chopped
1 dessertspoon olive oil
1 clove garlic, pressed or finely
chopped
2 teaspoons paprika
Splash of apple juice
Salt & pepper to taste
200g dry weight of cracked wheat (if
not available in your supermarket
use bulgar wheat instead)*

1. Firstly put on a pan of water to boil for the cracked wheat. Once the water is boiling add the cracked wheat and leave to simmer for 15 minutes. Then switch off the heat but leave to sit for a further 10 minutes before straining and rinsing with boiling water from the kettle.

2. In the meantime, in a large frying pan or saucepan heat the olive oil and add the onions. Cook until the onions are translucent which will take approximately 5 minutes. Stir regularly so they do not stick or burn.

3. Add the garlic, paprika and tomato purée, splash of apple juice and mix through thoroughly. Then add the can of tomatoes and season with salt and pepper.

4. Leave to simmer for 5 minutes, then add the mussels and leave to simmer for another 5-10 minutes to ensure they are heated through properly.

5. Once the cracked wheat is cooked, drained and rinsed, plate up and spoon the mussels in tomato sauce over the cracked wheat and serve.

Smoked Oysters in Tomato Sauce on a bed of Linguine IR, AC (for AC replace the linguine with whole wheat spaghetti)

Serves 1

1 small can smoked oysters, drained
1 small can tomatoes (preferably chopped or you can do this yourself)
1 tablespoon tomato purée
1 small onion, chopped
1 small chilli, deseeded & chopped (optional)
1 small splash olive oil
1 clove garlic, pressed or finely chopped
1 teaspoon paprika
Splash of apple juice
Salt & pepper to taste
100g dry weight of linguine

1. Firstly put on a pan of water to boil for the linguine.

2. In the meantime, in a large frying pan or saucepan heat the olive oil and add the onions. Cook until the onions are translucent which will take approximately 5 minutes. Stir regularly so they do not stick or burn.

3. Add the garlic, chilli (if using), paprika, tomato purée, splash of apple juice and mix through thoroughly. Then add the can of tomatoes and season with salt and pepper and simmer for 5 minutes.

4. Add the linguine to the boiling water. This should cook in 5-8 minutes dependent on the variety you are cooking.

5. Add the oysters to the sauce and leave to simmer for a further 5 minutes whilst you are draining and rinsing the linguine with boiling water.

6. Plate up the linguine, pour over the oyster and tomato sauce and serve.

Pan Fried Salmon IR, AC

Serves 2

2 fillets of salmon
1 tablespoon olive oil
Sweet chilli sauce (optional) Please
note this is not suitable if you are
following the Anti – Candida Plan

1. Remove any skin from the salmon with a knife. Check for and remove any obvious bones.
2. Wash the salmon under cold running water and then pat dry with kitchen paper.
3. Heat the oil in a frying pan. Wait until the oil is very hot before adding the salmon.
4. Leave it to sear for 4-5 minutes, depending on the size of the fillets. Then turn over.
5. Let the salmon cook for another couple of minutes. To check if it is cooked, gently use a knife and fork to prise open the flakes and see that the fillet is cooked all the way through.
6. *OPTIONAL:* Once the fillets have been turned, drizzle a little sweet chilli sauce over the top whilst the fish finishes cooking. It will warm the sauce and make a sticky coating over the fish. Serving suggestion: Serve with a rice noodle salad in the salad section.

Poached Salmon IR, AC

Serves 2

2 salmon fillets
A little oil
1 lemon, sliced
Some fresh fennel &/ or rosemary

1. Make a parcel for the salmon with some tin foil. Tear off a strip of tin foil, large enough to enclose the salmon, but to leave a space above it to allow the air to circulate in the parcel.
2. Pour a little oil onto the base of the foil to prevent the salmon from sticking. If the salmon fillets have skin on them, place them skin side down onto the foil.
3. Arrange the lemon slices over the salmon and then place the fresh herbs on top.
4. Pour in a drop of white wine or some stock, just to create a little moisture. It only needs to be a couple of tablespoons.
5. Seal the parcel and bake at 190C/375F until the fish has changed colour and is opaque. Depending on the Size of the fillets, this can take 20-30 minutes.

Herby Baked Trout IR, AC

Serves 1

1 fresh trout, gutted and cleaned
2 wedges of fresh lemon
Handful of fresh herbs of your choice
ie: tarragon, parsley, coriander,
rosemary
Drizzle of olive oil

1. Ensure the fish is clean and dry.

2. Make a parcel for the salmon with some tin foil. Tear off a strip of tin foil, large enough to enclose the trout, but to leave a space above it to allow the air to circulate in the parcel.

3. Pour a little oil onto the base of the foil to prevent the trout from sticking.

4. Put the lemon wedges and fresh herbs in the cavity of the trout.

5. Seal up the parcel by folding and rolling the tin foil. Bake at 190C/375F until the fish has changed colour and is opaque. Check after 15 minutes, but depending on the size of the fish, could take up to 30 minutes to cook.

Tuna Pasta IR, AC

(for AC use a whole wheat pasta, bulgar wheat, barley cous cous or brown rice)

Serves 2

150g can tuna, drained weight 100g

400g can tomatoes (preferably chopped or you can do this yourself)

2 tablespoons tomato purée

1 medium onion, chopped

1 dessertspoon olive oil

1 clove garlic, pressed or finely chopped

2 teaspoons mixed dried herbs

Salt & pepper to taste

200g dry weight of pasta of your choice

1. Firstly put on a pan of water to boil for the pasta.

2. In a large frying pan or saucepan heat the olive oil and add the onions. Cook until the onions are translucent which will take approximately 5 minutes. Stir regularly so they do not stick or burn.

3. Add the garlic, mixed herbs and tomato purée and mix through thoroughly. Then add the can of tomatoes.

4. Leave to simmer for 5 minutes

5. Once the water has come to the boil, add the pasta. This should cook in 8-10 minutes, depending on which variety you have chosen.

6. Add the tuna to the tomato sauce and stir through. Leave to simmer on a gentle heat.

7. Once the pasta is cooked, drain and rinse with boiling water from the kettle. This removes excess Starch and prevents the pasta from becoming sticky.

8. Season the tuna sauce, then add the pasta and stir through until it is coated in the sauce.

Tuna Bake IR

Serves 2

150g can tuna, drained weight
100g
400g can tomatoes (preferably
chopped or you can do this yourself)
2 tablespoons tomato purée
1 medium onion, chopped
1 dessertspoon olive oil
1 clove garlic, pressed or finely
chopped
2 teaspoons mixed dried herbs
Salt & pepper to taste
200g dry weight of pasta of your
choice
100g grated cheese

1. Firstly put on a pan of water to boil for the pasta.

2. In a large frying pan or saucepan heat the olive oil and add the onions. Cook until the onions are translucent which will take approximately 5 minutes. Stir regularly so they do not stick or burn.

3. Add the garlic, mixed herbs and tomato purée and mix through thoroughly. Then add the can of tomatoes.

4. Leave to simmer for 5 minutes

5. Once the water has come to the boil, add the pasta. This should cook in 8-10 minutes, depending on which variety you have chosen.

6. Add the tuna to the tomato sauce and stir through. Leave to simmer on a gentle heat.

7. Once the pasta is cooked, drain and rinse with boiling water from the kettle. This removes excess Starch and prevents the pasta from becoming sticky.

8. Season the tuna sauce, then add the pasta and stir through until it is coated in the sauce.

9. Put the pasta into an ovenproof serving dish and sprinkle the cheese on top. Either put the dish under a grill until the cheese is melted and bubbling. Alternatively pop into a moderate oven for a few minutes until the cheese is melted and browned.

Garlic Fried Seafood on Basmati Rice IR, AC

Serves 2

1 pack of mixed seafood from the supermarket chiller cabinet — contains prawns, mussels & squid
1 onion, peeled and chopped
1 tablespoon olive oil
2 cloves garlic, pressed
Small carton passatta
1 teaspoon dried mixed herbs
Salt and pepper to season
200g brown basmati rice

1. Put a saucepan of salted water on to boil. When it comes to the boil add the basmati rice and cook for approximately 10 minutes.
2. Heat the olive oil in a pan and add the onion and pressed garlic. Cook for a couple of minutes until the onion is softened, but take care not to burn the garlic.
3. Add the drained seafood, mixed herbs and passatta. Stir and allow to simmer for a few minutes until the seafood is piping hot. Season to taste and serve on a bed of basmati rice with a side salad of your choice.

Puy Lentils with Oven Roasted Vegetables & Goats or Feta Cheese IR, AC

Serves 2

125g Puy lentils cooked as per instructions or 1 pouch of microwavable Merchant Gourmet Puy Lentils
2 red onions, peeled and chopped into large chunks
12 cherry tomatoes
1 sweet potato, peeled and chopped into chunks
2 tablespoons olive oil
2 cloves garlic, thinly sliced
100g cheese of your choice, cubed
Juice of ½ lemon
Handful of flat leaf parsley, chopped
Sea salt and pepper to season

1. Preheat the oven to 180c.
2. Put the onions, sweet potato and cherry tomatoes onto a baking tray.
3. Pour over the olive oil and add the garlic slivers. Mix thoroughly so everything is coated in oil.
4. Bake in the oven for 25-30 minutes until the vegetables are soft.
5. Either cook the puy lentils whilst the vegetables are baking, or microwave the pouch of lentils.
6. Add the lentils to the vegetables and mix through. Sprinkle the cheese on top.
7. Return to the oven and bake for a further 5-10 minutes until the cheese starts to melt.

Thai Chick Peas IR

Serves 2–3

400g can chick peas, drained and rinsed
400ml can coconut milk (I used light milk to reduce fat content)
1 tablespoon rapeseed or olive oil
1 red onion, peeled and thinly sliced
200g sugar snap peas or mange tout
200g baby corn
1 red pepper, deseeded and sliced
1 red chilli, deseeded and chopped
1 thumb size piece of fresh ginger, peeled and grated
50ml apple juice
Small handful of chopped coriander
Salt and pepper to season

1. Heat the oil in a large pan. (I use a heavy based wok style pan).

2. Cook the red onion for a couple of minutes until is starts to soften.

3. Add the sugar snap peas, baby corn, red pepper, garlic and chilli and cook for a further couple of minutes, stirring all the time to ensure the garlic does not burn.

4. Add the ginger and apple juice, bring to the boil and allow it to simmer on a high heat for a couple of minutes.

5. Add the coconut milk, bring to the boil and allow it to simmer for 15-20 minutes to allow the milk to reduce and thicken.

6. Just before serving, season to taste and add the chopped coriander.

7. Serve with bulgar wheat cous cous or on a bed of brown basmati rice.

This dish can be made up to a couple of days in advance before serving. Ensure that the dish is stored in a covered container in the fridge.

Spicy Bean & Goats Cheese Cannelloni IR

Serves 2

410g can of Bean Cuisine (or mixed beans) drained & rinsed
1 stick celery
1 medium onion
1 red chilli – deseeded & finely chopped
Salt & pepper
1 tablespoon olive oil (use chilli oil for extra kick!)
Splash of Toasted Sesame oil (optional)
75g soft mild goats cheese (I use one with added garlic & herbs)
6-8 Cannelloni tubes (uncooked)
75g grated cheese
1 oven proof dish

Sauce

1 tblspn tomato purée
350g passatta (½ of a 700g jar)
1 clove garlic pressed or chopped
1 teaspoon dried mixed herbs
Salt & pepper

If you do not like your food spicy, just omit the red chilli.

1. Preheat the oven to 180c.
2. Finely chop the celery & onion.
3. In a frying pan, heat the olive oil, then add the celery, onion & chilli and cook for approximately 5 minutes until softened but not browned.
4. Add the drained and rinsed beans and cook for a further 5 minutes, stirring constantly until the beans are heated through.
5. Take off the heat and purée with either a hand blender or in a food processor.
6. Add the goats cheese and mix in thoroughly.
7. Put the bean mixture into a piping bag and fill each cannelloni tube. This mixture should fill 8 average sized cannelloni's. If you prefer, use half or two thirds of the mixture filling cannelloni's and reserve the rest for a dip to serve with crudités for a snack. (It should keep in the fridge for a couple of days). Put the filled cannelloni's into the oven proof dish.
8. In a saucepan mix all of the sauce ingredients together and heat, stirring occasionally. Once the sauce is bubbling, pour it over the cannelloni's in the dish.
9. Finish off with grated cheese and bake for approximately 30 minutes or until you can see the sauce bubbling and the cheese is browned.

Quesadilla IR, AC

Serves 2

2 Tortillas (see recipe provided)
1 buffalo mozzarella, drained and sliced
1 beef tomato, sliced, or 2 plum tomatoes, sliced
1 red onion, peeled and thinly sliced
1 handful fresh basil, roughly torn
2 tablespoons olive oil
2 tablespoons apple juice

1. Heat 1 tablespoon olive oil in a saucepan and add the red onion. Cook until the onion is softened then add the apple juice and simmer until most of the liquid has evaporated. Set aside.

2. Heat 1 tablespoon olive oil in a large frying pan. When hot put in 1 of the tortillas. Arrange the buffalo mozzarella on top of the tortilla, followed by the tomato, then the onion and finally the basil.

3. Put the other tortilla on top and carefully flip the quesadilla over to cook the other tortilla.

4. Once the mozzarella is melted and the quesadilla is browned, it is ready to serve.

5. With a sharp serrated knife, cut the quesadilla into 4. Serve 2 slices on a plate with a salad of your choice.

Pancetta Stir Fry with Broad Beans & Sugar Snap Peas IR, AC

Serves 2

6 thin slices pancetta
350g broad beans, either fresh or frozen
50g sugar snap peas
1 clove garlic, pressed
2 tablespoons olive oil
½ tablespoon lemon juice
Small handful fresh mint, chopped

1. Grill the pancetta on both sides until crisp. Set to one side.

2. Bring a pan of water to the boil and cook the broad beans for approximately 3 minutes. Throw in the sugar snap peas for approximately 30 seconds, then drain all of the beans immediately and refresh with cold water.

3. In a bowl, whisk together the garlic, olive oil, lemon juice and mint. Add the beans and arrange on serving plates. Lay the pancetta slices on top.

4. You may choose to serve this salad with homemade chapattis.

VEGETABLES

Roast Vegetables IR, AC

A selection of vegetables of your choice such as red, yellow, orange or green peppers, yellow, red or white onions, sweet potato, courgettes, to name but a few.
Olive oil or vegetable oil
2 cloves of garlic, peeled and cut into thin slices
2 teaspoons dried mixed herbs or some fresh rosemary, sage, thyme
Salt & pepper to season

1. Prepare your chosen vegetables by peeling and washing where necessary. Chop into chunks and ensure the vegetable are thoroughly dry.
2. Preheat the oven to 180c.
3. Put the prepared vegetables on a baking tray.
4. Drizzle over some oil, add the garlic and mix with your hands.
5. Put on some salt and pepper and sprinkle over the dried herbs or lay the fresh herbs on top.
6. Bake the vegetables for 25-30 minutes until golden and soft.
7. Remove the fresh herbs if used and serve.

Beans with Lemon & Pistachio Nuts IR, AC

Serves 2

250g French beans
50g pistachio nuts
2 tbsp olive oil
Zest and juice of ½ a lemon
Salt and freshly ground black pepper

1. Cook the beans in boiling, salted water for 3-4 minutes. Drain.
2. Remove the pistachio nuts from the shells and chop. Heat the oil in a pan and fry the nuts and lemon zest for 1-2 minutes.
3. Add the lemon juice and the beans and toss well to coat. Season to taste.

Sticky Red Onions IR, AC

Serves 2

2 medium –large red onions, peeled and thinly sliced
1 tablespoon olive oil
50ml apple juice

1. Heat the oil in a saucepan and sauté the onions for 2-3 minutes until they soften.
2. Add the apple juice and bring to the boil.
3. Leave the onions to simmer gently, uncovered for 45 minutes – 1 hour until they are soft and sticky.

Butter Bean Mash IR, AC

Serves 2

1 400g can butter beans, drained
and rinsed
3 tablespoons olive oil
3 tablespoons water
1 clove garlic, pressed
Juice ½ lemon
Small handful mint leaves, roughly
chopped (optional or change the
herb according to the dish)
Salt and pepper to season

1. Put all of the ingredients into a saucepan, bring to the boil and simmer for 10 minutes.
2. Put the ingredients into a food processor or blend with a hand blender.
3. Season to taste before serving.

Fennel & Butter Beans or Cannellini Beans IR, AC

Serves 2

1 bulb fennel
1 400g can butter beans (or
cannellini beans), drained and rinsed
2 tablespoons olive oil
Juice of 1 lemon
Small handful of flat leaf parsley,
finely chopped
Salt & pepper to season

1. Trim the fennel and remove the outside layer if woody. Thinly slice.
2. Heat the oil in a pan and add the fennel. Cook for a couple of minutes, stirring regularly until the fennel starts to soften.
3. Add the butter beans and lemon juice to the fennel and cook until the butter beans are heated through. Stir occasionally to prevent the fennel and butter beans sticking.
4. Add the flat leaf parsley, season to taste and serve.

SNACKS

Popcorn IR, AC

Serves 1

50g corn kernels

"Pop" the kernels in a popcorn maker. Alternatively, put the kernels in a microwavable bowl with a lid and cook on high for 2-4 minutes, depending on the wattage of your microwave.

Note: Please be careful of any unpopped kernels as they can be extremely hot.

You may choose to flavour your popcorn with a little salt, but do be careful how much you use!

Hummus IR, AC

Use either the recipe under the dips section, or use shop bought hummus. Just check to ensure that it does not contain disallowed ingredients.

Snack Size Sushi IR, AC

Available in many supermarkets. Do not use the soya sauce, pickled ginger or wasabi if you are following the Anti Candida plan. You can always add a drop of lemon juice if need be.

Roasted Spiced Nuts IR, AC

Serves 4

225g mixed nuts such as pecans, almonds, cashews & brazil nuts. DO NOT use peanuts due to mould.
2 tablespoons olive oil
¼ teaspoon chilli powder
¼ teaspoon garam massala or curry powder of some description

1. Heat the oil in a frying pan and fry the nuts for 2-3 minutes until they are golden.
2. Transfer the nuts to a bowl and sprinkle over the spices. Ensure they are tossed well to get an even coating.
3. Extra nuts can be stored in an airtight container for a few days.

Chapatis IR, AC

Makes 9–10

460g Spelt flour
½ teaspoon salt
275ml coconut milk or water
Oil for cooking

1. Put the flour and salt into a bowl and gradually add the milk (or water) until the mixture makes a soft dough.
2. Turn the dough out onto a lightly floured surface and knead until smooth (add more flour if necessary). Put the dough back into the bowl, cover and allow to rest for ½ hour.
3. Divide the dough into 9 or 10 balls and roll each ball out to approximately 6" (20cm) rounds.
4. Heat a heavy based frying pan and use sufficient oil to prevent the chapatis sticking. I like to use spray oil so you are not using too much.
5. Once the oil is hot, cook the chapatti for approximately 30 seconds to 1 minute each side (until bown spots appear).

Corn Tortillas IR, AC

250g Masa Harina (available in Sainsbury's &Waitrose)
330ml hot water
½ teaspoon salt

1. Mix all the ingredients together in a bowl to make a dough and let it rest for an hour.
2. Divide the dough into 10 balls and roll each ball out between 2 sheets of cling film or non-stick paper.
3. Heat the frying pan to a high temperature then cook each tortilla for 15 seconds each side, then 45 seconds each side and finishing with a further 15 seconds each side if necessary.
4. The tortillas can be made in advance if stored in an airtight container for 3-4 days.

ALTERNATIVELY, you can buy "AMAIZIN" Corn Chips, natural, organic & gluten free. I buy the 150g bags from the specialist food aisle in Sainsbury's.

Tortilla Dipping Chips IR, AC

1 egg white, lightly beaten
2 tablespoons olive oil
1 clove garlic, pressed
½ teaspoon chilli powder
½ teaspoon smoked paprika
3-4 corn tortillas

1. Preheat the oven to 180c.
2. Put all of the ingredients into a bowl (except the tortillas) and mix together.
3. Cut each tortilla into 8 pieces.
4. Brush one side of each tortilla piece with the egg mixture, the place on a baking tray.
5. When each tortilla piece has been prepared, bake in the oven for 5-10 minutes until crisp.
6. Transfer to a wire rack and leave to cool.
7. Any leftover tortilla chips can be stored in an airtight container for 3-4 days.

Iron Booster Bars IR

1 tbsp pumpkin seeds
1 tbsp sunflower seeds
1 tbsp sesame seeds
80g of chopped cashew nuts
25g chopped dates
25g chopped dried apricots
1 mashed banana
50g butter
1 tbsp golden syrup
½ tbsp molasses
25g soya flour
50g bran flakes
Juice of ½ lemon

1. Preheat oven to 180C / Gas 4. Grease & line a 7" round tin. If you double the quantity of the ingredients you can use an 18cm square tin.
2. Put lemon juice, syrup, molasses & butter into a saucepan, and heat until melted. Add the rest of ingredients and mix well.
3. Place mixture into tin, press down with the back of spoon and bake for 20-25 minutes until set and golden.
4. Remove from oven. Allow to cool in the tin and then cut into 8 bars. These bars store well in an airtight tin for a few days.

CHAPTER 11

Pregnancy and Hair Loss

It is generally a well known fact that during pregnancy, many women find that the condition and appearance of their hair improves dramatically. However post delivery they can go on to suffer diffuse hair loss which may last for a few months. This is due to the differing levels of hormones that pregnancy induces, prolonging the growth cycle of the hair. After delivery, oestrogen levels drop and more hair enters the resting phase, hence the increase in levels of hair loss.

I know I lost some hair after the delivery of each of my children. However, it was never enough to raise concern and it only really became apparent when the re-growth around the hair line kicked in and I realised how much hair I had actually lost!

If the hair loss you suffer after delivery goes on for an extended period of time and gives you cause for concern, consider the following:

1. Did you have a normal delivery?
2. Did you have to have an episiotomy?
3. Did you suffer second or third degree tears?
4. Did you have a caesarean section?
5. Did you have or were you offered a blood transfusion?
6. Were you given a course of iron tablets?
7. Did you have a blood test upon completion of a course of iron tablets?

If you suffered significant blood loss during delivery, it is possible that you may be anaemic or suffering from low iron levels. I was told I was anaemic after each of my three children's births and was given a course of iron tablets. However, after completing the iron tablets, I was never offered another blood test to check if my iron levels had been restored to an acceptable level. Hence, I assume that under my own circumstances, my iron stores depleted over a period of five or more years, culminating in a dietary deficiency causing the ultimate chronic shedding of hair.

I would suggest that if you are still suffering diffuse hair loss or alopecia areata more than six months after delivery, go back to your GP and ask to have your iron levels tested. Remember to ask for a serum ferritin test and if the level is under 40, this could well account for your hair loss. Should this be the case, read the chapters on low iron levels, the Iron Boost Food Plan, supplements for hair loss and the Anti-Candida Plan.

Please note: A lot of women suffer from heartburn and indigestion during pregnancy, due to the growing baby displacing or putting pressure on the stomach and digestive tract. If you need to take antacids (and I gobbled them like sweets!) try to wait two hours after eating a meal containing decent levels of iron. Iron binds with the calcium in antacids and will not be absorbed by the body. For this reason, also try to avoid consuming dairy products such as milk and cheese with iron rich meals.

CHAPTER 12

Stress and Hair Loss

When one of the Doctors I first spoke to about my alopecia areata told me to "take a break from the kids and do a yoga class", I found the advice to be most patronising. Now that I have a greater understanding of how stress impacts on hair loss, I can understand why this recommendation was made.

In most cases of alopecia, the patient will be asked if they have been exposed to a severe shock or a high degree of stress over the past few months. Many patients will admit to a degree of stress in their lives, but can then go on to recall much more stressful situations in their past, which have not resulted in hair loss.

It can also be extremely annoying as a patient to be asked this question. When your hair is falling out by the handful and it appears to be everywhere around you except on your head, you are going to feel stressed!

Combine this with the lack of a definitive prognosis and treatment plan which is often the case with diffuse hair loss and alopecia areata, it can often serve to enhance the degree of stress and before you know it, you can add depression to your list of ailments.

To combat this, you have to work at removing or dealing with the stress in your life. Firstly you have to understand why it can affect your hair loss.

When stress is applied to our body in either a physical or mental form, the body has to do it's best to protect itself. If this occurs over a prolonged period of time, hair is an obvious target to shut down, as it is not essential for survival. Chemicals are released which instructs hair follicles to prematurely enter the telogen (resting phase) of the hair cycle.

Unfortunately this disrupts the hair growth cycle. Despite the normal shedding taking place within the next two to four months, all the additional hair that was resting will not only fall out, but the new growth will not have occurred to take its place. This will result in the thinning of hair.

If you are not careful the condition can be exacerbated by the very fact that you are suffering stress due to the excess loss of hair and you end up in a downward spiral of stress and hair loss.

It is also worth noting that chronic stress can reduce blood flow to the gut leaving it unable to repair itself, which in turn will have an impact on the effectiveness of the ability of the gut to absorb nutrients.

To resolve the situation you either have to remove the object of stress or, if this is impossible because you are dealing with the stresses of modern day life such as work, commuting, work/life balance etc, you need to take time out for yourself to relax. Yoga would be an excellent example of a beneficial activity to partake in, but as long as you are doing something that takes your mind off of your stress triggers and your body relaxes, you will be doing yourself some good.

Despite the above making sense, I do not fully subscribe to stress on its own being the cause of on-going hair loss, particularly in the form of alopecia areata. Over the years there have been studies conducted to substantiate this. I do still believe that it is possible for a sudden traumatic shock to result in more or less immediate hair loss. However, I believe that stress is a contributory factor working in conjunction with other physical problems and it may prove to be the final trigger that results in the shedding of hair.

CHAPTER 13

Diet and Hair Loss

I cannot begin to express my amazement at how little is attributed to the correlation between diet and hair loss. For one of the most logical factors to contribute towards hair loss, diet is so readily dismissed. Research in this area is improving and I understand that the Western diet *should* provide sufficient nutrition for optimum hair growth. However, we are exposed to a plethora of convenience foods which can be counter productive, if we become dependent on them to exclusively supply our dietary needs.

Healthy hair requires a regular intake of protein and a variety of vitamins and minerals to sustain good growth. A decline in the appearance of your hair and finger nails are often the first sign that nutritionally, all is not well with your diet.

We are currently living a world where a significant number of women suffer from iron deficiency, to such a degree that it can impact on their health. In the UK we all but pay lip service to the importance of iron in the diet of pregnant women. It would appear to only be considered a problem if the woman suffers anaemia and even then, it is often poorly managed after diagnosis.

In a world where to be a size zero equates to being put on a pedestal alongside skeletal celebrities, women and teenage girls are allowing their health to suffer by not eating sufficiently nutritious food.

Unfortunately it is a common fallacy that red meat is bad for you, alongside faddy diets that cut back on proteins and fats. To be healthy we need all food types (with the exception of sugar) in our diet. We just have to learn to consume them in the correct proportions.

This is made additionally harder with all the convenience foods readily available. In the Western world we are becoming more dependent on food manufacturers to fortify foods with nutritional supplements, which ironically have often been removed in the processing of them!

A lot of the land that our food is grown on has been over-farmed during the past 50 years, resulting in a lower nutritional value of the produce, as the soil becomes exhausted. Again, we need to be aware of this fact in order to ensure that we are consuming sufficient unprocessed foods and maybe even take supplements, to ensure our optimum nutritional requirements are obtained.

Once again, if you exercise aerobically on a regular basis, please ensure you are meeting your additional nutritional requirements. It is no coincidence that distance runners are now being advised to keep track of their iron levels.

As I have mentioned before, I am convinced that the catalyst for my own chronic hair loss was caused by a combination of already very low iron stores being depleted through an insufficient iron intake in my diet, coupled with the impact of a strenuous exercise regime causing further depletion, during a ten week weight loss programme.

CHAPTER 14

Medication (prescription or otherwise) and Hair Loss

There are some medications that can cause/contribute to hair loss. Most people will be aware of the effects of Chemotherapy drugs, but there are many other drug treatments that can influence hair loss. If you should fall into this category, your Doctor may already be aware of the side effects of your medication, however there are some drugs that can be overlooked, so I will just mention the ones that I know about.

It is also worth noting that hair loss due to medication is generally diffuse hair loss / excessive shedding. However, I did discover a link between alopecia areata with certain forms of antibiotics/penicillin.

Thyroid

If you are receiving medication for either an over-active or under-active thyroid, it is possible that your hair loss may be linked to the medication that you are taking, as well as being a symptom of the condition. Check with your Doctor that hair loss is not listed as a possible side effect.

Synthroid is well known to cause hair loss for an underactive thyroid and Carbimazole for an over active thyroid.

The Pill

If your hair loss started after commencing the pill or changing your pill medication, it is possible for this to be the cause. All oral contraceptives use progestogens (synthetic hormones) to replicate the effect of progesterone. Unfortunately some are not as good as others. If you are taking any of the following oral contraceptives norgestrel, norethisterone or levonorgestrel, and this coincides with hair loss commencing, ask your Doctor to change you to another medication.

Anti Depressants

If you have been prescribed any of the following forms of anti depressants, they may account for the onset of hair loss. Prozac, Paxil, Zoloft, Amphetamines.

Thrush

If you regularly suffer from Thrush and self medicate with over the counter preparations, you may be suffering from hair loss caused by the active ingredient in the medication. In addition, if you suffer from Thrush, I suspect you may also have candida of the gut which may be the ultimate cause of your hair loss. I would strongly recommend following the Anti-Candida Plan which may also help to treat further flare ups of Thrush.

Hay Fever Medication

It was brought to my attention last year that several of the over the counter Hay Fever remedies can result in hair loss. Within a short time of taking a well known brand of the non drowsy variety, my mother started to shed hair. Fortunately she recognised the hair loss had been triggered by the medication and when she checked the information leaflet, hair loss was cited as a possible side effect. I did wonder if this was a contributory factor towards my hair loss during the first summer of my hair loss. Further investigation revealed that many of the hay fever medications do mention hair loss as a possible side effect, particularly the non-drowsy varieties. Last year I used Piriton and did not suffer any side effects.

Statins Medication

Statins are drugs prescribed to help reduce cholesterol levels in those of us suffering from high cholesterol. Unfortunately a side effect can cause hair loss. As statins are generally taken for life, I was very sceptical about taking them when my GP suggested I should, due to my elevated cholesterol level. I have endeavoured to reduce my cholesterol levels through diet and exercise. Although statins would undoubtedly reduce my cholesterol levels further, I, along with my Doctor, considered the possible detrimental effects to outweigh the benefits in my case.

Accutane

Accutane is used for the treatment of severe acne. Some sufferers can experience hair loss within a few days of taking the drug. Some people may experience hair loss after completing a course of Accutane and therefore, may not be aware of the possible connection. Hair loss caused by taking Accutane can be temporary or permanent. Therefore do check with your Doctor if this medication has been prescribed for you.

In addition to the drugs mentioned so far, the following conditions can be treated with drugs that may cause hair loss: HRT, different forms of steroids, weight loss tablets (amphetamines), anti-coagulants (Warfarin), Ulcer Medications (Zantac), Heart/High Blood Pressure Medications and treatments for Gout.

In view of this extensive list, do ask your Doctor to check the details of any medications prescribed, as it is possible that an alternative treatment may be available, if indeed your prescription could be the cause of your hair loss.

CHAPTER 15

Trichodynia — Hair Pain / Scalp Pain / Pony Tail Syndrome

This is yet another symptom/condition that I suffered during my battle with hair loss. My hair loss cycle was already well established when I suffered my one and only attack of what is sometimes referred to as Trichodynia, but is more readily identified as scalp pain.

Trichodynia struck sixteen months after the first patches of alopecia areata appeared. I had suffered a bout of chronic hair shedding, followed by a further five months of alopecia areata. The scalp pain first started in August 2007. At this time my hair, although still short had been recovering well. Remaining patches were filling in and I was feeling reasonably good about myself. The initial scalp pain started with a "pony tail" sensation. The feeling you get when your hair has been pulled tightly in a pony tail for too long. The problem was my hair was too short to even contemplate a pony tail! This went on for a couple of days and started to get progressively worse. The tightness of the scalp turned into a painful sensation from which there was no relief. With it came feelings of impending doom.

Within a week of the first sensations becoming established, I was taking paracetamol before going to bed. Just laying my head on the pillow became extremely painful. I hoped it would pass, but instead I started suffering from other symptoms. For no apparent reason I would suddenly get "crawling" sensations on my scalp, as though an army of bugs were on a march, weaving in and out of my hair follicles. I became paranoid that I had picked up head lice, despite my husband's assurances to the contrary. To add insult to injury, I started to get raised angry bumps all over my head which were incredibly itchy, yet to scratch them was impossible as my scalp hurt so much.

Once again I looked on the internet and found threads of discussions where dozens of women all over the world were describing the same symptoms as me. They also received little if any help from their Doctors. I decided not to go to my Doctor with these symptoms as I was concerned that I would be considered a nuisance. Instead I decided to wait until my scheduled appointment in September, but by then the symptoms had disappeared, only to be replaced with the onset of my worst attack of alopecia areata.

In some ways I consider myself fortunate, as I have only experienced one attack. Many women suffer from Trichodynia on a regular basis, yet it was only officially recognised as a condition during the mid nineties. Very little research has been conducted into the condition, but a tentative link has been made between

Trichodynia and diffuse hair loss. In fact, the term Trichodynia is not yet recognised with a definitive dictionary definition.

One study detailed in the International Journal Of Dermatology (Volume 42, Number 9, September 2003, pp. 691-693(3)) concluded that Trichodynia is a common symptom in patients with Telogen Effluvium (diffuse hair loss) and Androgenetic Alopecia (male pattern baldness), and often coexists with psychopathologic findings, including depression, obsessive personality disorder and anxiety.

Although I am unable to comment on the obsessive personality disorder, I would suggest that it stands to reason that people suffering from any form of hair loss, are quite likely to suffer from depression and anxiety! What was not made clear was whether the conditions were in place before the hair loss occurred, or were a result of the hair loss.

Unfortunately I am not in a position to offer any advice on how to treat this condition. I have seen a couple of shampoos for sale on the internet in the USA which uses capsicum (a variety of tropical pepper plants) to block Substance P (the body's pain messenger). I have been unable to establish whether there is any credence to the claims.

CHAPTER 16

Hair Loss – a symptom of Environmental Illness?

I have suspected for a while that hair loss, whether it be Alopecia Areata or Telogen Effluivium is a symptom of another illness as opposed to a disease in its own right. My research has uncovered evidence to support this, albeit in slightly different formats. Before I go on to these in more detail, I must first explain what an Environmental Illness is.

Currently there is not one agreed definitive definition of what constitutes an Environmental Illness. However, it is loosely agreed to refer to a patient suffering symptoms that are directly linked to and triggered by the environment in which they live. Currently chronic fatigue syndrome (ME), fibromyalgia, irritable bowel syndrome, candida, leaky gut syndrome, gulf war syndrome and autism have been classified as Environmental Illnesses. In addition, these patients usually present a history of allergies and sensitivities which have been a part of their life for many years. These can include asthma, hay fever, multiple contact sensitivities and allergies as well as food sensitivities and allergies.

From my own personal experience, in the past I have been diagnosed with chronic fatigue syndrome, fibromyalgia, candida and leaky gut syndrome. Yet when I followed an anti-candida diet for 6 weeks, all of the symptoms disappeared! The second time I suffered different symptoms in the form of alopecia areata, diffuse hair loss and symptoms of hypothyroidism (even though I was not diagnosed with the condition). Once again, the symptoms were resolved through following an anti-candida plan.

It has been discovered that many patients who suffer from poor absorption of iron are also found to be deficient in other minerals as well, such as zinc and selenium. These two minerals are required to produce an enzyme which is essential for the healthy functioning of the thyroid hormones. The T3 hormone is responsible for getting every cell in the body to use more oxygen and for all the tissues to produce proteins. Without T3 working properly, everything in the body slows down producing the symptoms of hypothyroidism.

In addition it is known that candida produces a toxic chemical called acetaldehyde, which in severe cases can accumulate in body tissues and prevent T3 getting into the cells. This could explain why thyroid blood tests come back as normal due to the body producing the correct hormone levels, but this hormone is being blocked from functioning correctly.

Dr Jacob Teitelbaum of the Fibromyalgia & Fatigue Centers, Inc. (FFC) treats patients suffering from environmental illnesses such as chronic fatigue syndrome (ME) and fibromyalgia with a thyroid treatment. His protocol has been subjected to controlled clinical trials in which its effectiveness was verified and he has helped thousands of people to recover from their illnesses. When I found Dr Jacob Teitelbaum's research, I wondered if it was applicable to me and if so, perhaps my hair loss was the result of the combined effect of a faulty thyroid, low ferritin levels and candidiasis.

I then discovered further research with amazing results conducted by Dr. Michael McNett, President and Medical Director of The Paragon Clinic in Chicago, USA. His clinic specializes in treating fibromyalgia and muscular pain. Dr McNett has discovered that many fibromyalgia patients also present symptoms of hypothyroidism, despite having normal blood test results for the condition. He also found that they tend to test positive for candida hypersensitivity syndrome. Once the candida is treated, the hypothyroidism symptoms generally disappear.

Could this mean that hair loss is yet another symptom of environmental illness? After all, Alopecia Areata is known to be an autoimmune disease. Therefore, should the treatment of hair loss in general take a more holistic approach? This line of investigation would surely be more beneficial to the patient because not only are they "doing" something to see if it will improve or cure their hair loss, it could also rid them of a host of other symptoms, which may have been regarded as irrelevant to their hair loss in the past.

As this book goes to press, I am currently helping a woman who has been suffering from Alopecia Areata for a few years. She has also been plagued with chronic Irritable Bowel Syndrome for nine years. I suggested she should start on the Anti-Candida Plan as soon as possible, which she did.

"Within the first week most of my IBS symptoms had disappeared. I am currently in my seventh week of the plan and this is my third consecutive week completely free of IBS symptoms". Emma

It is still too early to see if the plan has helped her Alopecia Areata, but for this young woman to be able to function normally just by changing her diet, surely indicates that candida requires further investigation.

CHAPTER 17

Practical tips for day to day life whilst suffering hair loss

Don't feel a fraud

I can recall several occasions when my alopecia was at its worst and I was wearing hats in an attempt to disguise it, feeling guilty that people had misinterpreted my hair loss as being the result of chemotherapy. In retrospect, this was entirely unnecessary on my part. Although you may feel okay physically, the psychological effects of alopecia areata can be devastating.

I recall having a conversation with a lady who supplied beautiful head wraps, as I needed something a little more elegant than a baseball cap for my husband's office party! She dealt with a lot of women suffering hair loss due to the side effects of chemotherapy and was very sympathetic. However, when I weighed up what the majority of her clients were facing against my hair loss, I felt that I had no right to complain.

With alopecia, because the cause of hair loss is unknown, the sufferer never knows if and when their hair will grow back. The pattern of my alopecia was very frustrating as I would go through a "grow back" phase and just when I had achieved a full head of hair again, regardless of how short it was, patches would start appearing again in different areas on my scalp.

Be proactive about supporting yourself

This is the time when you need to use the support of family and friends.

If, for example you are a mum making regular trips to the school playground, make sure that you mention to other mums that you are suffering from alopecia. The known playground gossips are often a good one to target, as you are guaranteed to get your news in full circulation! I found it really helped to "get the truth out there" and chat to friends and acquaintances alike. This will dispel any suspicions on their part as to what is the cause of your hair loss and also helps them to overcome their embarrassment or discomfort whilst in your company.

Once again, if you find this too difficult to do yourself, engage your family and friends to help.

Ask a couple of family members or friends if you can nominate them as a person that you can "sound off" to. So that on those occasions when you feel really down, you can vent it to them, as this can really help you work through the emotional side of the condition.

I found it better to use someone who may not be as emotionally attached as a close family member, as this can be distressing for them too and you may not fully let go of what you are feeling, in an attempt to protect their emotions too.

Don't Let Yourself Go!

Fitness
This was one of the biggest regrettable mistakes I made.

Comfort eating and drinking can turn into yet another result of suffering from alopecia areata. In addition, I stopped doing my regular exercise and yoga classes, because I was too embarrassed to go to a gym. I was acutely conscious that if I participated in yoga, where you often have your head down, any headgear I was wearing would slide off. What a mistake as yoga and pilates are a fantastic way to not only exercise the body, but also to release tension in the mind and help you to relax. However, I have since found that Luscious Lids have recently added a new head cover called a Cotton Interlock Turban, which tightly covers the whole head, but is also cool. It is also available in 60 different colours!

I stopped swimming with my children where in retrospect, it didn't even occur to me to buy a swimming hat!

If you really cannot face a public place of exercise, invest in some home work-out dvds. Yoga and pilates are excellent and if you need to raise the heart rate, there are dozens of dvds on the market where you do not need loads of space to work out. However, if you are wary about intensive exercise potentially triggering hair loss again, take up walking. I joined a walking group and found that once I had achieved a proper walking technique, my physique really improved. Plus, all you need to cover up is a baseball cap.

Whilst I was well on the way to recovering from my hair loss ordeal, I was still wary of strenuous exercise in case it should trigger hair loss again. Fortunately this coincided with my meeting Joanna Hall of "Walk Active" at a health & beauty show. After chatting to Joanna about my recent health problems she assured me that her style of walking would not only improve my fitness, muscle tone and aid weight loss, I would not lose any hair in the process. I took a leap of faith at this time and threw myself into her Walk Active programme. True to her word, within weeks I was looking and feeling so much better. At the three month stage I did get nervous, but fortunately no hair loss occurred. I went on to feature on the success page of Joanna's website (www.joannahall.com) and also completed the 2010 London Moonwalk of 26 miles, all thanks to her understanding and encouragement. Joanna, I cannot thank you enough to get me over that last hurdle and ultimately get back to being "me" again.

Finally, if you work at improving your fitness, you will release those powerful endorphins which will not only make you feel better in yourself, but will also help to curb any food cravings and resultant comfort eating.

Your relationship with food

If you are one of those people who cannot face food whilst feeling down, remember that this could exacerbate your condition.

Telogen Effluvium (extreme shedding of hair) I believe in my case, was triggered by a strict vegetarian diet accompanied by intensive exercise for a period of 10 weeks. My protein intake was lower than I required plus my diet also meant that I had a low iron intake. As, unbeknown to me at the time, I was running on very low iron stores anyway, this transpired to be a critical combination which ultimately instigated this phase of my hair loss. It is essential, particularly when you are losing hair, in whatever guise, that you ensure you are supplying your body with the necessary building blocks with food and supplements, to aid recovery.

It is pertinent to mention at this point, that long distance runners are now advised to ensure that they are receiving optimum levels of iron in their diet as they tend to excrete it whilst training.

If on the other hand you become food dependent, always reaching out for something to give you that quick sugar high, you are also potentially exacerbating the condition. A diet which is full of sugars and refined carbohydrates have the potential to affect your progesterone levels, which in theory, can affect your hair growth, as well as potentially aid the growth of candida albican in your gut.

As I have already identified in the chapter relating to Candidasis, this is far more likely to have an effect on your overall health and hair loss is likely to be a symptom.

Appearance

Loss of hair can really influence how you feel about the rest of your appearance. I felt like a sexless object for a while and just wanted to hide myself away. Fortunately having a young family, this was not possible in my case, so I had to deal with how I was going to face the outside world.

Keep any skincare and beauty regime you had before losing your hair and where possible, add to it. After all, if you are not spending lots of money on hairdressing bills, invest the money in yourself in other ways. Treat yourself to manicures, pedicures, massages, facials etc. If you like make up, purchase some new eye colours to give your eyes a more dramatic look or buy a more daring shade of lipstick.

Ask for a makeover at any of the major cosmetic counters in department stores and tell the Consultant why you want their help. A sympathetic Beauty Consultant may also indulge you in some extra samples to try at home! If you are unfortunate enough to have lost your eyebrows and/or eyelashes, there are many ways to overcome this now. A good beautician should be able to show you how to pencil in realistic looking eyebrows. You may even consider having them tattooed if you have suffered from long term hair loss. There are also many varieties of false eyelashes available now. It just takes practise and a little trial and error to learn how to attach them in place.

Hair

As for your hair, even if you don't have a lot, indulge what you have!

I chose to invest in aloe vera shampoo and conditioner from a health food shop. Price wise it was comparable to many commercial brands on the market and I also felt reassured that I was not causing further damage with unknown chemicals in the shampoo formulations. I have since tried shampoo and conditioner from Culpepper the herbalist as well as Wish Hair Care. (details in the Suppliers List).

I have naturally dry hair and the aloe vera products certainly improved the feel and appearance as well as being gentle on the scalp. As were the ginger and hemp products from Culpepper. Unfortunately, they no longer appear to be available. Finally the Passionflower & Chamomile Shampoo and Rosewood & Bergamot Conditioner by Wish Hair Care make my hair feel soft and luxurious at a reasonable price. It is really important to consider your scalp as usually a good layer of hair will protect it. I can remember one summer when I was in a "grow back" phase, having two patches on the top of my head, which got sunburnt one sunny afternoon. Not a pleasant experience! Therefore, don't forget to have sunscreen or wear a hat.

Hats

This leads me nicely on to the topic of hats. I now have loads of hats, summer, winter, casual and formal. Anything from a baseball cap to dressy wide brimmed one for a wedding.

Also, don't panic about the price! There is a very well known high street store that likes to turn over stock cheap and fast. For my cousin's wedding I bought a wide brimmed felt hat and finished it by tying a cream (which matched my jacket) silk scarf around it. No one at the wedding had any idea that I was disguising stubble for hair underneath, and it only cost me a tenner!

The biggest challenge I had was my husband's office Christmas Party. I had to come up with a suitable head covering to suit a trendy Notting Hill restaurant where we had to "dress to impress". Fortunately I found a brilliant website on the internet called "Luscious Lids". The lady makes headwraps in all different designs and colours using a variety of fabrics. I ordered a wrap in black velvet which is secured with two long ties which can be wound and intertwined together in a variety of ways, to secure the wrap to your head. I chose the second tie to be in a contrast colour. Because natural fabrics are used your head does not sweat and it gave me a real confidence boost going out in it.

In addition, when everyone sat down for dinner, there were a variety of crazy party hats to wear, so I did not stand out during the evening as being the only person wearing a head covering!

Again, I would like to point out that at £18, this was not an expensive purchase and it was used several times over the festive period.

Wigs

Unfortunately this is one area where I cannot offer much advice from experience. Although it was suggested to me that I should buy a wig, it was an area where I felt extremely disadvantaged. My natural hair colour is red and because it is a unique shade, there is no way it could be replicated with a wig. Therefore, I felt that if I went out in a wig, people who knew me would know that I was wearing one and this would make me feel self conscious. However, if I was blonde or brunette, I would probably have considered it.

If you do decide to go down the wig route I can offer a couple of tips passed to me by my hairdresser (she used to cut and style wigs for clients). Surprisingly she recommends buying synthetic over human hair. Apart from the obvious cost saving, they are a lot easier to look after. A human hair wig has to be treated like real hair when it comes to washing and styling. A synthetic wig is cut into a style and it stays in that style. General rule of thumb is it should be washed every fifteen to twenty wearings, with the cleaning solution provided, although this will vary with heat, humidity etc as it would with your own hair.

The other tip is to have your wig cut and thinned. This can seem a bit scary if you have just invested a lot of money in a wig. After all, the hair is not going to grow back! However, the style needs to be cut to suit your face shape and to reflect your personality. In addition, it needs to be thinned out by approximately 30% to rid it of that "wiggy" look!

For further information I suggest looking at this website www.mynewhair.org, a charity which is run by Trevor Sorbie. In addition to being an excellent hairdresser, he has been involved with the use of wigs for many years. He is also very understanding of the plight of women whom have lost their hair and offers a free consultation. Not everybody is able to get to see Trevor Sorbie himself, but there is a list of participating salons up and down the country that subscribe to his wig fitting service. In addition, there are lots of other details and advice regarding the purchase, fitting and wearing of wigs.

Wigs are available on the NHS but I believe the prescription has to be written by a Dermatologist and you must be either bald or have suffered significant hair loss for a year or more. You may also be means tested to see if you can contribute toward the cost.

Hairdresser

One of the biggest problems facing a hair loss sufferer is finding a hairdresser who is sympathetic to your condition and who can look after your needs. I was extremely lucky in that I have a friend who was a hairdresser for many years and has had experience with styling people whom have suffered from alopecia, as well as fitting and styling wigs.

This meant that I could have my hair cut by someone that I knew and trusted, in the comfort of my own home, without having to worry about invasive looks from strangers.

Perhaps you are lucky enough to have a good relationship with a long standing hairdresser that you trust. If not, you may wish to try and track down a local mobile hairdresser. Usually someone can be recommended by word of mouth and this way you do not have to get stressed out worrying about being head naked in a hairdressing salon.

Hair Colouring/ Hair Treatments

In Beckenham, Kent, The Organic Hair Salon uses fabulous products for hair in general as they use completely natural products, which contrary to popular belief, hold the same depth of colour as more conventional colours. They are also very sympathetic towards clients dealing with hair loss, so if possible, they are well worth a visit.

Diary or Blog

It may help you to keep a record of your experiences whilst suffering from hair loss. It certainly helped me to write this book! I would also suggest having photographs taken at regular intervals for your reference. This is something that I did not do, as particularly when my hair was at its worst, I hid from the camera. Now I wish I had a fuller record so that I could share my journey through pictures as well as words.

If you choose to Blog, you may well link up with other hair loss sufferers and be able to support each other.

Getting back on your feet

Once that magical re-growth appears and establishes itself, it is time to let go of the past and look to the future. As my confidence had taken a knock and I had hidden myself away for so long, I challenged myself to "get out there" again. I did this by auditioning for a television programme "Britain's Best Dish" and managed to get selected to cook in the studio. Unfortunately my dish did not go down so well with the Judges on the day, but I thoroughly enjoyed the whole experience, particularly making new friends, none of whom had any idea that only a few months earlier, I was practically bald!

Secretly plan yourself a "coming out" date. Make it a date within the coming weeks or months, when you will feel confident about re-launching yourself again. Sometimes a birthday, a family occasion or a party will give you a date to work towards, not only regarding your hair, but your overall look. If your confidence has taken a knock it will give you time to maybe lose those extra pounds gained through comforting yourself with the biscuit tin! You can look forward to buying a new outfit, getting an updated make up look and getting in shape physically. As long as whatever you choose to do will make you feel better, then indulge yourself, you deserve it!

CHAPTER 18

Useful contacts / suppliers for women suffering from hair loss

Please note: The following information was correct going to press, however changes may well occur.

Food

This is where I purchase the more "out of the ordinary" foods mentioned in the eating plans. It is not to say that they are not available in other stores.

BARLEY COUS COUS – specialist food section in Sainsbury's.

COCONUT OIL – I have used the organic coconut oil which I purchased over the internet. However, I found coconut oil for sale in a larger Sainsbury's store at a fraction of the price of the organic version and it was just as good.

LINSEED OIL – High Barn Oils, Muntham Home Farm, Barns Green, Horsham, West Sussex, RN13 0NH. Tel: 01403 730 326. www.highbarnoils.co.uk.

MERCHANT GOURMET PUY LENTILS – these come either in microwavable pouches, canned or in boxes, uncooked. I have purchased them in Sainsbury's and Waitrose.

MARIGOLD STOCK CUBES – available in all major supermarkets.

COLD PRESSED RAPESEED OIL – I use 2 different oils, Hillfarm Extra Virgin Cold Pressed Rapeseed Oil which I have bought in Sainsbury's and Farringtons Mellow Yellow Cold Pressed Rapeseed Oil which I have purchased in Sainsbury's, Waitrose and from Ocado.

SAVOUR BAKES OAT NIBBLES – Aldi supermarkets.

Hairdresser

I am happy to recommend the following Hairdressers due to the sympathetic nature of their staff and also the natural hair colourants and products that they use.
The London Organic Hair Salon,
10 High St,
Beckenham, BR3 1AZ
Telephone: 020 8650 0555

Head Coverings

I cannot recommend Luscious Lids highly enough. If you place a telephone order you will receive plenty of advice on which fabrics to order, which head wraps are suitable for which occasion and in a large variety of colours. The service is

sympathetic, delivery prompt, quality excellent and great value for money too!
Luscious Lids
14 Briarswood Rise,
Dibden Purlieu,
Southampton, SO45 5SW
Telephone: 023 8084 8687
Email: sheila.wilson@lusciouslids.com
www.lusciouslids.com

Kinesiology
If you would like to find a practising Applied Kinesiologist near you, please go through the association and use a registered practitioner.
Telephone: 0845 260 1094 (9am – noon)
Web: www.kinesiologyfederation.co.uk

Shampoos & Conditioners
Wish Hair Care
By far the best natural hair care products I have tried. They produce shampoo and conditioner for all hair types and you can rest assured you will not be massaging any harsh chemicals into your scalp with their products!
www.beautifullygorgeous.co.uk

I have also used a variety of Aloe Vera hair products available in both health food shops and from Forever Living. Once again, they are using natural products so are less likely to cause scalp irritation and will be gentle on your hair.

Supplements
All of the following supplements are available at Boots, GNC, Holland & Barrett as well as local chemists and health food shops.

L-Lysine (500mg), Vitamin C (100mg), Zinc (15mg).
Magnesium OK or Magnesium B by Wassen are available in most high street chemists and health food shops.

Aloe Vera Juice
Please buy the sugar free variety only. Available at GNC, Holland & Barrett and Forever Living Products.

Acidophilus
The best capsules I have come across are from **BioCare.**
Telephone: +44 (0) 121 433 3427 Web: www.biocare.co.uk

Bio-Acidophilus Forte 30 Capsules. Catalogue code: 16130. Price: £26.65. Take 1 per day or Bio-Acidophilus 60 Capsules. Catalogue code: 16860. Price: £18.95. Take 2 per day.

Elemental Iron
I recommend the following iron capsules as they are gentler on the stomach than any iron tablets your GP would prescribe. Please double check with your Doctor that he/she approves the use of them in your case.

There are other Iron capsules available from BioCare, but they contain added vitamins at added expense. If you are already following the recommended supplements I have discussed, then there is no need to purchase these other capsules. Iron eap complex 60 capsules, catalogue code: 20260, price £8.00 (15mg).
Telephone: +44 (0) 121 433 3727
www.biocare.co.uk

Spirulina
Available in both powder and tablet form
Telephone: +44 (0) 1342 888098
www.microrganics-uk.com

Walking for fitness
I cannot recommend Joanna Hall's Walk Active Club enough. Joanna and all of her staff are truly devoted to the cause of using Joanna's walking technique to achieve optimum fitness and health benefits. Joanna's walking courses and time trials are available across the country. Even if you go for just one time trial to learn the walking technique, it will be well worth it!
www.joannahall.com

I also have to recommend Walk The Walk, the charity which runs the Moon Walks in the UK and now the Sun Walk too. Not only are you walking yourself to fitness by following the training schedules for the walking marathons, you are also raising valuable sponsorship money for breast cancer charities.
www.walkthewalk.org

Wig Stylists
Trevor Sorbie, celebrity hairdresser has set up a charity called My New Hair. The purpose of the charity is to assist people who have lost their hair, for whatever reason, to get their wigs fitted and styled. He has set up a network of salons which have all agreed to offer this service at a nominal or affordable fee. There is also plenty of further information available regarding hair loss.
www.mynewhair.org

CHAPTER 19

Bibliography

Clarke, Jane, 29 May 2007, "Red meat and two veg can beat hair loss" *Mail Online*.

Dodds, Rosemary, "Being vegetarian and eating right for your age" *Mail Online*.

Harvey, Graham, 2006, *We Want Real Food*. London: Constable.

McNett, Michael, *Candida and yeast and the connection to thyroid disease and fibromyalgia*. An interview with Dr. Michael McNett. www.thyroid-info.com/articles/candidayeast.htm.

Teitelbaum, Jacob, *Thyroid Treatments*,

www.ei-resource.org/illness-information/related-conditions/thyroid-treatments/

CHAPTER 20

Photo Gallery

Before hair loss

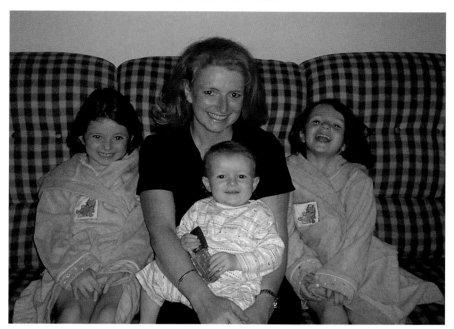

Summer 2004

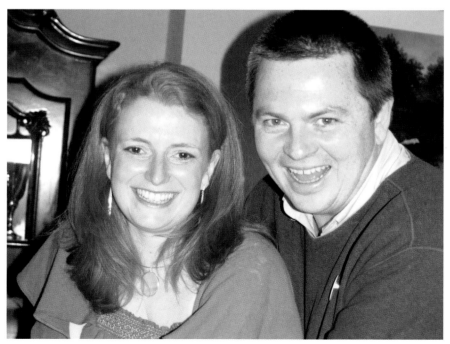

Spring 2005

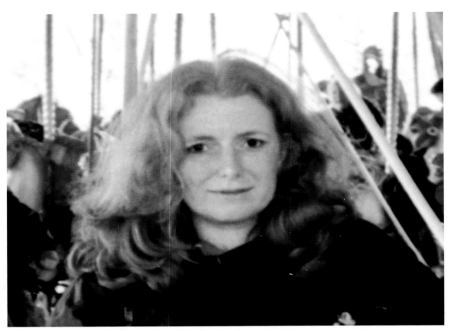

February 2006

During hair loss

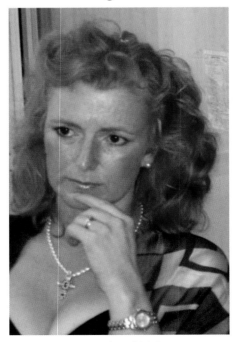

October 2006

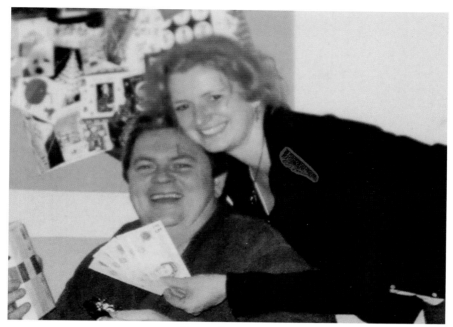

December 2006

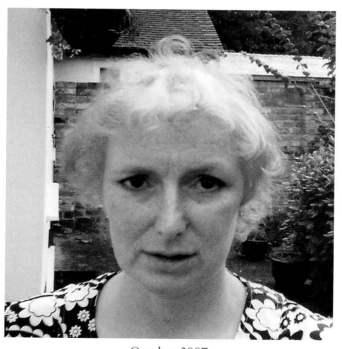

October 2007

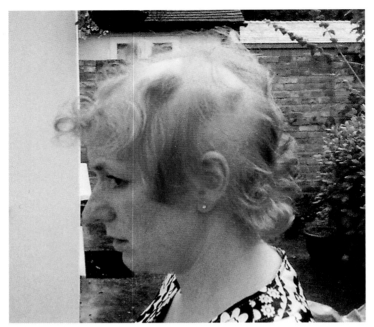

October 2007

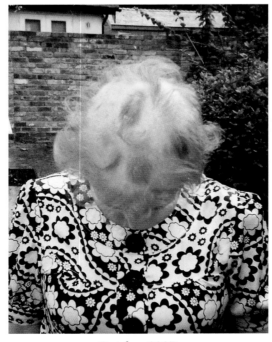

October 2007

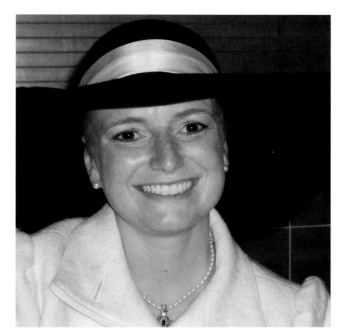

November 2007

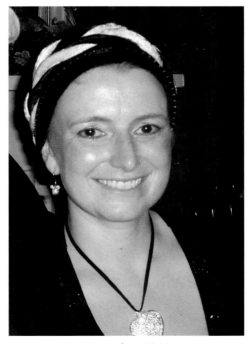

December 2007

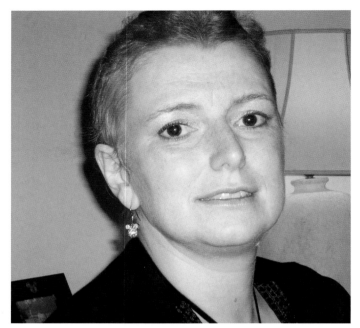

December 2007

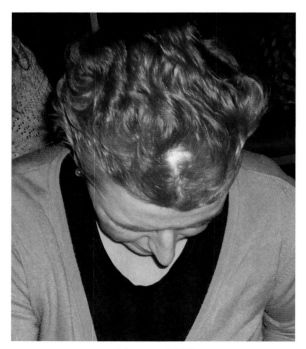

February 2008

After hair loss

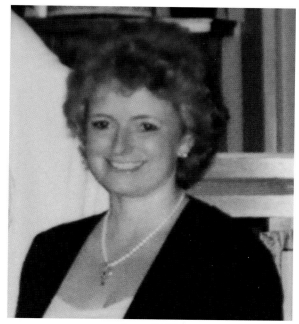

June 2008

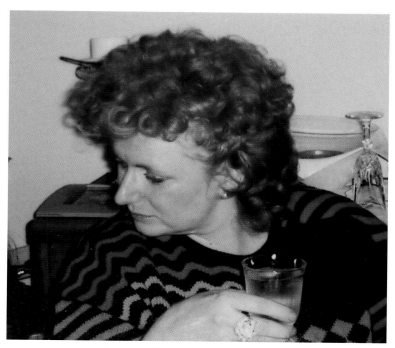

December 2008

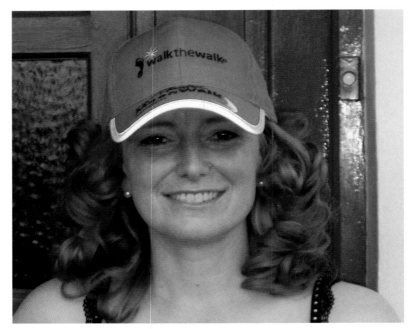

May 2010

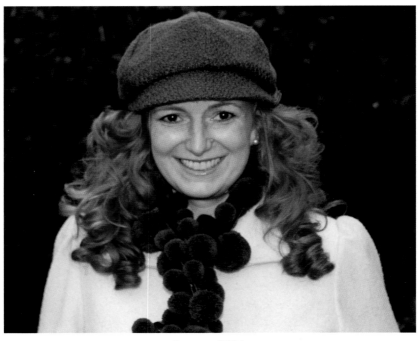

January 2011